DO YOU KNOW . . .

- How simple memory aids can make a big difference?
- How reality orientation helps people who are severely confused?
- What to try to relieve feelings of anxiety and nervousness?
- What is one of the best ways to handle wandering?
- What *never* to tell a person with Alzheimer's?
- Which strategies work best to maintain a balanced diet?
- How a social life is possible . . . and important?
- How an adult-day-care center can be a lifesaver . . . for both patient and caregiver?
- How to evaluate your own emotional state as a caregiver?
- What to do if you, the caregiver, get depressed or overstressed?

WHEN SOMEONE YOU LOVE HAS . . . ALZHEIMER'S

Dell Caregiving Guides

QUANTITY SALES

Most Dell books are available at special quantity discounts when purchased in bulk by corporations, organizations, or groups. Special imprints, messages, and excerpts can be produced to meet your needs. For more information, write to: Dell Publishing, 1540 Broadway, New York, NY 10036. Attention: Director, Special Markets.

INDIVIDUAL SALES

Are there any Dell books you want but cannot find in your local stores? If so, you can order them directly from us. You can get any Dell book currently in print. For a complete up-to-date listing of our books and information on how to order, write to: Dell Readers Service, Box DR, 1540 Broadway, New York, NY 10036.

The Dell Caregiving Guides

When Someone You Love Has Alzheimer's

Marilynn Larkin

Deborah Mitchell, Contributing Editor

Foreword by Allen D. Roses, M.D.

A LYNN SONBERG BOOK

Published by
Dell Publishing
a division of
Random House, Inc.

If you purchased this book without a cover you should be aware that this book is stolen property. It was reported as "unsold and destroyed" to the publisher and neither the author nor the publisher has received any payment for this "stripped book."

Research about Alzheimer's disease is ongoing and subject to interpretation. Although every effort has been made to include the most up-to-date and accurate information in this book, there can be no guarantee that what we know about this complex subject won't change with time. The reader should bear in mind that this book should not be used for the diagnosis or treatment of Alzheimer's disease and should consult appropriate medical professionals regarding all health issues.

Copyright © 1994 by Lynn Sonberg Book Associates

All rights reserved. No part of this book may be reproduced or transmitted in any form or by any means, electronic or mechanical, including photocopying, recording, or by any information storage and retrieval system, without the written permission of the Publisher, except where permitted by law.

The trademark Dell® is registered in the U.S. Patent and Trademark Office.

ISBN: 0-440-21660-5

Published by arrangement with Lynn Sonberg Book Associates, 260 West 72nd Street, Suite 6-C, New York, New York 10023.

Printed in the United States of America

Published simultaneously in Canada

November 1995

10 9 8

OPM

Acknowledgments

The author gratefully acknowledges the assistance of Allen D. Roses, M.D., who generously gave of his time and shared his groundbreaking research in Alzheimer's disease with her. She is also grateful to the staff of the Alzheimer's Association–New York City Chapter, who shared their expertise: Rea Kahn, Support Group Coordinator, and the members of her spouse support group; Anne Thomas, Home Care Aides Training Program Coordinator; Gail Hoffman, Volunteer Coordinator/Program Associate; and Jed Levine, Coordinator of Training and Special Projects. Special thanks to Deborah Mitchell for assisting in the research and preparation of this manuscript.

Contents

Foreword by Allen D. Roses, M.D. — xi
Introduction — xiii
    The Difficulty of Caregiving — xv
    How This Book Can Help — xvi

ONE **Becoming a Caregiver** — 1
    Deciding to Become a Caregiver
    Accepting Your Feelings
    The Grieving Process
    Revealing the Diagnosis
    After the Diagnosis: What to Expect

TWO **What You Need to Know About Alzheimer's Disease** — 18
    What Is Alzheimer's Disease?
    What Causes Alzheimer's Disease?
    How Is Alzheimer's Disease Diagnosed?
    What Are the Symptoms of Alzheimer's Disease?
    What Is the Treatment?

THREE	**Helping with Memory and Communication Problems**	30
	Memory Loss	
	Coping with Memory Loss	
	Memory-Related Communication Problems	
FOUR	**Helping with Mood and Behavior Problems**	45
	Anxiety and Nervousness	
	Wandering and Restlessness	
	Combativeness and Anger	
	Clinging Behavior	
	Depression	
	Hallucinations	
	Delusions	
	Paranoia	
	Hoarding and Hiding	
	Sexuality	
FIVE	**Helping with Physical and Personal-Hygiene Problems**	69
	Creating a Safe Environment	
	A Room-by-Room Safety Guide	
	Loss of Coordination	
	Incontinence	
	Constipation	
	Bathing	
	Dressing and Undressing	
	Grooming	
SIX	**Your Role in Medical Therapy**	101
	Selecting a Physician to Coordinate Care	

CONTENTS

Selecting Other Health Professionals
A Word About Lifestyle
Drugs: What Every Caregiver Should Know
Organizing Medicines
Managing Medical Problems
Other Medical Conditions
Hospitalization

SEVEN **Mealtimes and Nutrition**   131
Problem Eating Behavior
Problems with Chewing, Swallowing, or Drooling
Successful Mealtimes
Maintaining Good Nutrition
Menu Planning
Tips for Improving Nutritional Intake
Meal-Preparation Tips
Shopping Tips

EIGHT **Exercise, Socializing, and Other Activities**   151
Exercise Has Many Benefits
A Social Life Is Possible
Recreational Activities and Hobbies

NINE **When to Consider Other Living Arrangements**   167
Deciding to Get Help
Having Someone Come into Your Home
Adult-Day-Care Facilities
Foster Care

Life-Care Facilities
Nursing Homes
State Mental Hospitals
Hospices

TEN **Financial and Legal Concerns** 184
Finding Professional Help
Legal Matters
Financial Assessment

ELEVEN **Caring for Yourself** 201
Accepting Your Feelings
Paying Attention to Your Own Well-being
Taking Action to Relieve Stress
Take Care of Yourself: A Checklist

TWELVE **Resource Guide** 216

Glossary 231
Index 235

Foreword

Caring for a person with Alzheimer's disease requires emotional strength and stamina, courage, and fortitude. In a very real sense, the caregiver—spouse, child, sibling, other relative, in-law, friend—is as much a victim of the disease as the person who receives the diagnosis. Shock, denial, fear, depression, and feelings of rage or helplessness are common reactions to learning that a loved one has the disease; these feelings must be accepted and eventually overcome so that everyone involved can proceed with the familiar routines and new challenges of daily life.

When Someone You Love Has Alzheimer's Disease can serve as a guide and companion during this difficult time. This book presents practical strategies for helping with the many memory, communication, mood, behavior, physical, and medical problems that are symptomatic of the disease. In addition it offers advice on planning for the future—financial and legal considerations, as well as what to do when home care is no longer possible. A comprehensive chapter on resources enables the reader to contact numerous organizations—both national and local—that can offer in-depth help in all these areas.

Although this book clearly offers much-needed assistance to the caregiver today, it is my hope that in the future it will no longer be needed. Recently much research in laboratories around the world has led to major breakthroughs in our understanding of the possible causes of Alzheimer's disease. This new knowledge is leading to the development of better diagnostic tests and has pinpointed targets for new treatments and therapies to delay the onset of the disease and ultimately prevent it from developing. Today's caregiver may take comfort in knowing that although Alzheimer's disease is taking a toll on a spouse or parent now, there is every reason to believe that research will lead to the treatment and prevention of Alzheimer's disease in the future.

> Allen D. Roses, M.D.
> Jefferson Pilot Corp.
> Professor of Neurobiology and Neurology
> Chief, Division of Neurology
> Duke University Medical Center
> Durham, North Carolina

Introduction

Mary was engaged in one of her favorite activities—doing the crossword puzzle in the daily paper. "I don't know what's the matter with me," she said to her husband, Jerry. "The clue is ' "Blank" Velvet,' the name of a song. I know the first word is a color, but I can't remember what it is."

"Well, it's not as bad as forgetting the name of our mailman, which you did yesterday," Jerry teased. But beneath his teasing tone, Jerry was worried. Mary's memory lapses were occurring more frequently. Something was wrong with her, and that realization frightened him.

Mary is in the early stages of Alzheimer's disease, a devastating illness that ultimately leads the sufferer to a state of total dependence on caregivers. The most insidious aspect of the disease is that it begins almost imperceptibly; moments of forgetfulness, among the first symptoms, are easily attributed to distraction, emotional upset, or simply a "normal" part of aging.

But there is nothing "normal" about Alzheimer's. It is an organic brain disease that takes a tremendous toll on the person with the illness, the caregiver, and society at large. Currently more than four million Americans suffer from Alzheimer's. The prevalence increases dramatically with age. People age sixty-five to seventy-four have a one in twenty-five chance of having Alzheimer's; for those age eighty-five and older this likelihood rises to a staggering nearly one in two chance. This eighty-five-plus age group is the most rapidly growing sector of the American population, which means we may expect a dramatic increase in the overall number of people with Alzheimer's in the coming century, unless preventive treatments and cures are discovered.

Alzheimer's disease affects the cells of the brain, producing progressively severe intellectual impairment. At first the individual experiences only minor and almost imperceptible symptoms that may be attributed to emotional upset or other physical illnesses. The person may forget to turn off the oven, misplace things, recheck to see if a task was done, or repeat already answered questions. As the disease progresses, memory loss increases and other changes, such as confusion, irritability, restlessness, and agitation are likely to appear. Judgment, concentration, and speech may also be affected.

There are many different patterns in the type, severity, and sequence of changes in mental and neurological functioning that result from Alzheimer's disease. Although the symptoms are progressive, there is great variation in the rate of change from person to person.

During the early stages the person with Alzheimer's is likely to be aware that his or her mental faculties are becoming impaired. This realization can be agonizing to the person with the disease and may trigger depression and other mood changes. The decline may also have terrible emotional consequences for the spouse and children of the person with Alzheimer's, especially when they are the caregivers.

During the later stages Alzheimer's can cause complete dependency. The person with Alzheimer's may eventually lose the ability to walk and to eat and swallow, and may need round-the-clock care at home or in a nursing facility.

THE DIFFICULTY OF CAREGIVING

Caring for a person with Alzheimer's takes courage and fortitude. As the National Institute of Aging points out, the caregiving burden is not simply a matter of money, though care can be costly, especially when patients are repeatedly hospitalized during the course of their illness. In addition active caregivers, as well as family members and friends who take on part of the caregiving responsibilities, may suffer from depression, exhaustion, isolation, and increased health problems. For example, Peter told himself, "I've had it. Mom is getting worse and worse. I feel as though I can't stand the sight of her anymore. Then I feel guilty." Peter eventually decided to ask his sister to share in caregiving so that he could take some much-needed time for himself.

If you are a caregiver, you may be reluctant to ask for help, feeling that the person with Alzheimer's is your responsibility or that you must be stoic and handle everything yourself. These are mistaken beliefs. All caregivers can benefit from support from others and from the practical information contained in resources such as this book. No one has to "go it alone."

HOW THIS BOOK CAN HELP

This book can help you in three very important ways. First, *When Someone You Love Has Alzheimer's* lets you know that you are not alone in your feelings, frustrations, and difficulties. No matter how much you may love a person with Alzheimer's, there will be times when you lose patience or feel distraught, angry, and helpless. This book will help you understand that such feelings are perfectly normal, and not a cause for guilt or self-recriminations.

You'll also learn how others like yourself use specific techniques to help the person with Alzheimer's live as full a life as possible through each stage of the disease. This book contains practical strategies for dealing with the stressful symptoms of Alzheimer's, including memory loss, behavior problems, and physical dysfunction, and explains the roles of proper nutrition and exercise in helping to lessen the severity of some symptoms.

Finally, this book provides suggestions for ensuring your own health and well-being by asking for help from others. It also gives you important information about financial and legal planning for the future.

Chapter 1 covers your role as a caregiver and describes the many responsibilities you will need to undertake during the course of the disease. You'll also learn what to expect after a diagnosis of probable Alzheimer's disease is made.

Chapter 2 answers the most commonly asked questions about Alzheimer's disease, including how it is diagnosed, the symptoms, and treatments that may help alleviate symptoms. It also covers the steps entailed in enrolling the person with Alzheimer's in studies to test experimental treatments.

In chapter 3 you'll learn strategies for coping with the memory and communication problems that can be among the most difficult for caregivers to handle. Techniques will include the use of memory aids, exercises to help the person stay oriented in the environment, and strategies to improve communication skills, which are often affected by memory loss.

Chapter 4 presents techniques that help alleviate mood and behavior problems. You'll learn how to reduce the person's feelings of depression, anger, or listlessness; how to handle suspiciousness and hallucinations; how to respond to combative or inappropriate behaviors such as clinging, making constant demands, losing or hoarding things, and repetitive actions.

Chapter 5 offers strategies for helping with physical problems so that the person with Alzheimer's is as safe and comfortable as possible in the home and community. Physical aids that assist in maintaining balance and coordination are covered. Techniques for helping with personal hygiene and incontinence are also addressed.

Chapter 6 covers your role in helping to manage the person's medical problems, such as vision, hearing, dental problems, and pain. Medications that are sometimes prescribed to treat symptoms are covered. This chapter also contains a section on selecting a physician and other health professionals who are experienced in caring for people with Alzheimer's disease, and what to do if hospitalization is required.

Chapter 7 covers the importance of good nutrition in helping to reduce the severity of certain symptoms. Meal planning and preparation tips are offered, as well as information on helping with eating and swallowing.

Chapter 8 discusses the benefits of exercise, socializing, and other activities in helping the person with Alzheimer's make the most of his or her remaining years.

Chapter 9 provides guidelines for making other living arrangements, such as a nursing home or other long-term care facility, when appropriate. The types of facilities available and tips for evaluating them are discussed.

Chapter 10 covers the financial and legal issues you must consider when the person for whom you are caring can no longer handle these matters. Concepts such as power of attorney and living wills are discussed, as well as other documents you will be asked to complete on the other person's behalf.

In chapter 11 you'll learn strategies for coping with the emotional and physical stresses of caregiving so that you can stay healthy and avoid burnout.

Chapter 12 is a Resource Guide that includes names, addresses, and phone numbers of organizations to contact for more help and information.

Remember, caregivers around the country and around the world face many of the same problems and experience many of the same feelings that you do. You are not alone, nor should you be.

By trying the strategies suggested in this book, communicating with knowledgeable health professionals, and securing appropriate support when needed, you will succeed in providing the compassionate care a person with Alzheimer's needs to preserve as much happiness and dignity as possible during the course of this devastating illness. You will also be in a better position to preserve your own health and well-being during this painful process.

ONE

Becoming a Caregiver

"I really couldn't believe this was happening to Harry. At first, when he started to forget things, we just joked about it. Then one day we were in the car and he forgot how to get to the mall—or back home. That's when I started getting nervous. I couldn't deny there was a problem—and neither could Harry. I knew he wanted to make light of it, but he couldn't find the words. Later we talked about it. I suggested we go to the doctor, and Harry resisted the idea. A few days later I had our daughter come over and talk to him about it again. He finally agreed to go. It was a wrenching experience—so many tests, no one wanting to say anything definite. But a few weeks later our doctor called me with the diagnosis."

—Shirley

"This disease is something we all dread. And when Helen was diagnosed with probable Alzheimer's, I nearly fainted. The hard part was telling her. She wasn't very far gone, and she was devastated. We didn't know what to do, and we both kind of panicked. Should we tell our sons and daughters? Did we really have to worry, since she seemed pretty okay? Suddenly the future looked very grim. Our doctor recommended that we talk to someone at the Alzheimer's Association, and that helped put

us on the right track. We told our family and they're being very supportive. We may not have a lot to look forward to, but at least we'll try to enjoy whatever time we have."

—Sam

"At first I thought I could handle taking care of Mom, since she lived nearby, and my sister lived hours away. Well, it worked out all right the first year of Mom's illness, when she wasn't too disoriented. But then she began to decline very rapidly. Sometimes she didn't know who I was, refused to change her clothes, and really couldn't take care of herself at all. I had to call my sister and insist we arrange to take care of Mom together. I was overwhelmed. I felt so angry at Mom, and helpless. My husband complained I was spending all my time over there, and coming back too tired to pay attention to our family. When my sister hemmed and hawed, I exploded. 'If you don't help,' I said, 'then I'm not doing anything.' I just couldn't go on, it was so painful. Well, she did end up helping, and eventually we put Mom in a nursing home. We visited every day and made sure Mom was as comfortable as possible. Last month, she passed away."

—Diane

Being a caregiver for a person with Alzheimer's disease is a difficult, often heart-wrenching job. Since the disease has a course from two to twenty years, it's impossible to know from the outset how long the job will last, but regardless of the duration, caregiving is likely to consume your time, sap your strength, and trigger many strong emotions. You may end up neglecting many aspects of your own life—job, friends, family, leisure activities—as you focus increasing amounts of time and energy on the needs of the person with Alzheimer's.

In this chapter we'll cover the factors that go into the decision to become a caregiver and your responsibilities over the course of the disease. We'll also review the kinds of changes you can expect the person with Alzheimer's to undergo, and introduce you to some of the health professionals who can help you during the process.

DECIDING TO BECOME A CAREGIVER

Many caregivers don't have an opportunity actually to decide to undertake the job of caring for a person with Alzheimer's. In effect the caregiving role is foisted upon them by circumstances, such as when the person with Alzheimer's is a spouse. On the other hand a son, daughter, or other concerned relative who is not living with the person may need to sit down with members of his or her own family and figure out how to fit caregiving into the rest of his or her responsibilities. This may mean sharing the caregiving role with other relatives or friends, or seeking professional assistance. The organizations listed in chapter 12 provide information on health care, insurance, caregivers' support groups, and free or low-cost services that can make caregiving easier.

Some people are reluctant to become caregivers because, like Roger, they worry whether they are capable of doing the job. "I never had to cook or clean, much less take Heline to the bathroom. Sure, she doesn't need me to do that now. But the doctor said down the road it's going to happen. If I start taking care of her now, what will I do then?" Roger said.

It really doesn't matter whether you have previously nursed a sick person or not. You can still be a caregiver, learning as you go and having the comfort of knowing that you are doing the best job you can possibly do. What's more, if you become accustomed now to admitting when some aspects of caregiving are too much and asking for help, by the time more difficult tasks arise, you will have supportive helpers—other family members, friends, neighbors, professionals—in place.

ACCEPTING YOUR FEELINGS

The Alzheimer's caregiver is often called the hidden victim of AD. While the physical effort of caregiving may result in exhaustion, sleeplessness, or even physical injury, the emotional stress can cause anger, tension, guilt, depression, anxiety, and feelings of helplessness, worthlessness, and fear. Moreover you will feel grief—grief for the loss of the person you knew as personality changes and changes in the relationship take place—often for years before the person's death.

Caregivers often find that their feelings shift and change over the course of the disease. In the early stage denial—pretending symptoms are simply something to joke about, as Shirley and Harry did—is the most common feeling, since accepting the reality of Alzheimer's means accepting a difficult future. As the disease progresses, you may feel many of the other feelings described above, such as helplessness, fear, and depression. If you hesitate to reach out for help, you may become increasingly isolated and lonely. If other family members are affected by the person's disease, you may have to deal with their emotions as well.

Because your feelings, when not accepted or appropriately expressed, can cause harm to you and, by extension, to the person you're caring for, it's very important to acknowledge your emotions and accept them as part of a natural reaction to the caregiving process. Joining an Alzheimer's support group or finding a concerned listener who is not intimately involved in your situation—a social worker, clergyman, or other professional—is crucial to your well-being.

THE GRIEVING PROCESS

Because, at this writing, Alzheimer's disease is inevitably fatal, you are likely to experience strong feelings of grief and loss from the outset if the person you are caring for has been someone close to you. As the disease progresses, you will find yourself grieving for the person you knew as a loving spouse, parent, or other close friend or relative. Dealing with these feelings is also part of the caregiving process.

The grieving process has been described in stages. These stages are neither inevitable nor necessarily sequential. One stage doesn't abruptly stop so that the next can begin. You may move back and forth among the stages at your own pace. And although "coping" is the last stage, you will certainly be coping with the situation to some extent throughout the process.

Stage 1: Shock

"I must be dreaming. This can't really be happening to us!"

Feelings of numbness, unreality, confusion, helplessness, and fear may be experienced by the caregiver and the person who has received an Alzheimer's diagnosis. The support of family and friends is crucial at this time.

Stage 2: Denial

"I don't care what the doctor says. Henry looks fine and feels fine. So he forgets things occasionally. So do I."

Denial is the way we avoid facing the overwhelming reality of a devastating situation. Although it permits you to cope for a time, eventually you will have to face the truth and start taking steps to prepare for the future.

Stage 3: Reaction

"Our lives are destroyed. Nothing will ever be the same."

When you begin to accept the reality of Alzheimer's, depression often sets in. Some people feel so distraught that they believe immediate death would have been preferable to living with the inevitable decline they now face. This is a very normal reaction; do not feel guilty about feeling this way. It is part of the grieving process.

Other common reactions, which may go hand in hand with depression, are anger and frustration.

"I thought, 'How could Alice do this to us? We had our whole retirement set—vacation, new home near the kids. And now she gets sick!' I know it sounds ridiculous, but I blamed her for her illness. I couldn't help myself."

Again, these feelings are normal—not a cause for guilt or self-recrimination. The important thing is to move through this phase into acceptance. Only after mourning the loss of the person he or she knew can a caregiver learn who that person has become and begin to develop a comfortable relationship. It is a slow process that is difficult for all concerned.

Stage 4: Mobilization

This is the action stage, when the caregiver, and hopefully the person with Alzheimer's as well, begin to switch their focus from the problems they cannot control to the ones they can control. Learning about available resources, doing financial planning and health care planning, and taking other steps to make the course of the disease easier are all helpful during this stage.

Stage 5: Coping

This is the stage in which caregivers become more realistic about their abilities and how much they can do, and also become realistic about the changing abilities of the person they're caring for. You can enjoy reminiscing about the past while recognizing that the person has very different needs and abilities now.

"I take each day at a time and try to get something positive from it. At the same time I prepare for the future."

Remember, there are no set time limits for any of these stages. You reach the coping stage when you are ready—and even then you may move back into earlier stages for brief periods. Respect your feelings and allow yourself to grieve and heal at your own pace.

REVEALING THE DIAGNOSIS

By the time a diagnosis of Alzheimer's disease is made, most people know that something is wrong with them. How much they need to be told will depend on how far the disease has progressed and how much they want to know. Many already suspect "the worst" and may even have been trying to cover up for memory losses or problems with doing daily tasks. Revealing the diagnosis acknowledges that a disease is responsible for the difficulties he or she may have been experiencing.

Be honest with yourself about your ability to tell the person about the diagnosis. If you feel you will need help, consider asking your physician to talk with the person while you are present, or have another close friend or relative with you.

Also answer the person's questions honestly. Reassure the person that you love and support him or her. Explain that you will help make plans for the future.

You and the person with Alzheimer's will also need to tell other family members about the diagnosis in order to enlist their help and understanding. Be aware that others may have reactions ranging from disbelief to shock and fear. Many will also undergo a grieving process similar to the one that you will experience.

Explain that some of the behaviors the person displays now or in the future are those he or she cannot control. Encourage others to extend their love and help to the individual and ask them to support you in your role as caregiver.

"I didn't know how anyone in the family would react when I told them Quinn had Alzheimer's," Darlene said.

"Our son and daughter were extremely supportive and offered to fly right in. My sister acted as if it were something contagious and never visits anymore. That hurts, especially when Quinn asks where my sister is. I always make excuses for her, but I think he knows the reason. Quinn's brother visits quite a bit, but I can see he's wondering if he's going to get it too."

Dealing with your own feelings, the feelings of the person with Alzheimer's, and the reactions of family and friends can be a very trying experience and will require a great deal of emotional strength on your part.

AFTER THE DIAGNOSIS: WHAT TO EXPECT

Once a diagnosis of Alzheimer's disease is made, you and the person with Alzheimer's are likely to experience the shock and denial that are hallmarks of the grieving process, described above. At the same time you must begin dealing with the reality of the disease and start planning for the future. Knowing what to expect as the disease progresses can help you prepare for the consequences.

How quickly the disease runs its course and the types and extent of impairments that result may vary greatly from person to person. Eventually, however, Alzheimer's disease leaves the person totally unable to care for himself or herself. On average Alzheimer's lasts about eight years; however, it may last as little as two years or as long as twenty years.

During this time, changes in the individual's personality, changes in relationships, and physical and emotional exhaustion are the most common areas of concern for the caregiver, whether spouse, child, sibling, friend, or other relative. Following is an overview of what to expect in the days, weeks, months, and years after a diagnosis of Alzheimer's disease. These concerns, and strategies for coping with them, will be addressed in detail in the following chapters of this book.

Personality Changes

Alzheimer's inevitably changes the established behavior patterns that we associate with an individual's personality. Some of the more common personality changes due to Alzheimer's disease include demanding, unreasonable, and combative behavior. Other symptoms may include confusion, disorientation, poor judgment, and language problems.

Relationship Changes

After a diagnosis of Alzheimer's disease, relationships undergo many changes and therefore can be a source of tremendous stress. Adult children may find themselves functioning in a parental role to their own parent, or a spouse may find himself or herself functioning as a parent. The person with Alzheimer's may feel the helplessness and dependency often associated with childhood, especially in the early stages when he or she is aware of the onset of impairments. He or she may feel unattractive and fear the rejection of loved ones. Sexual relationships will change. These changes are difficult for all concerned.

Physical and Emotional Fatigue

Meeting the needs of a person with Alzheimer's disease requires an extended commitment of physical and emotional effort. New demands will be made on your time and energy, which you must meet in addition to the old ones. It can be very difficult to juggle all these responsibilities, and you may begin to feel pulled in too many directions at once.

To take some of the pressure off, remind yourself that you are human, have limitations, and can only try to do your best. By taking an occasional break from caregiving you will give yourself an opportunity to take stock, relax, and refuel. This is vital for you and for the person for whom you are caring. No caregiver can function effectively and give to others if he or she is exhausted or burdened by a sense of unreasonable guilt.

Your Responsibilities as Caregiver

As a caregiver for a person with Alzheimer's you face many challenges. Unfortunately as of now there is no cure for the disease, though researchers are optimistic that much progress will be made in the next few years. In the meantime you are charged with making the remaining years of the person with Alzheimer's as comfortable and productive as possible. At the same time it is important for you to enjoy your own life as much as possible as well.

Your caregiving responsibilities will be determined primarily by the course of the disease. In fact you may not have fully adjusted to one stage of the disease before the second stage sets in and a whole new set of difficulties emerges.

It is imperative that the person with Alzheimer's be under a physician's care from the outset. Advice on selecting an appropriate physician and other health professionals can be found in chapter 6.

In the early stages, when the person with Alzheimer's has relatively few symptoms, your responsibilities include being attentive to the person's needs, mitigating memory or communication problems (see chapter 3), and staying alert to changes in the person's condition (see chapter 6). You should also schedule regular visits with a physician and other health professionals. Another important step is commencing financial planning, including the execution of a living will and assignment of durable power of attorney, and applying for whatever benefits the person may be entitled to (see chapter 10).

In the middle stages of the disease, depending on the degree of impairment, you may also need to adapt your home for convenience and safety (see chapter 5). Sometimes medications are prescribed to help with some of the symptoms of Alzheimer's, such as depression, or preexisting medical conditions such as hypertension. You will need to monitor and possibly help manage the medication schedule (see chapter 6). You will also be coping with the changing personality of the person with Alzheimer's and possibly beginning nursing and custodial duties (personal hygiene, use of the commode). By now you should also be actively participating in legal and financial decision making.

During the later stages of the disease your responsibilities may include being as attentive as possible to needs that can no longer be expressed, maintaining the medication schedule, arranging for an alternative living situation (see chapter 9), making plans for what will happen after death, and saying good-bye to the person in your own way.

Essential Caregiving Skills

The essential skills you will need during this process include the following:

- Good organization. You will need to keep track of medical, legal, and financial records, medication schedules, and schedules of others who are available to assist you in caregiving.
- Physical stamina. You may need to lift and carry the person with Alzheimer's, deal with custodial duties, and go without a regular sleep and meal schedule.
- Emotional stamina. You will need to deal with your own feelings toward the person with Alzheimer's, as well as that person's feelings and the feelings of other family members and friends. You will also need to be able to distance yourself occasionally from these intense and often contradictory feelings in order to function.
- The ability to deal with boring, repetitive, and often distasteful jobs. In the early stages of the disease you may be involved in exercises to help slow the decline of memory and speech; in the middle and later stages much of the work you will do revolves around food, elimination, and personal hygiene.
- The ability to manage the rest of your life, protect your own health and well-being, and make peace with death and dying.

Your Team of Health Professionals

In addition to supportive family, friends, and support-group members, it is important to enlist the assistance of your physician and other health care professionals to provide optimal care to the person with Alzheimer's. An overview of some of the key professionals you may be working with is presented here. The skills of some of these professionals often overlap (for example, nurses and occupational therapists are both trained in helping with activities of daily living), so that you may not need the services of every type of practitioner listed here. Advice on selecting a physician and other health professionals is presented in chapter 6.

Physician

Since Alzheimer's disease can last up to twenty years or more, it is important to select a physician you like and trust to coordinate the person's care. This can be your current family physician or another physician experienced in the care of people with Alzheimer's disease.

Nurses

Nurses can teach you how to handle bathing, eating problems, and transfers; help you address behavior problems; teach you how to administer medications and use special devices, such as shower seats or wheelchairs; and give you suggestions on how to make your home environment safe.

At some point you may want to have a visiting nurse in your home. Ask your physician for recommendations, or contact your county home health agency or the Visiting Nurse Association. Depending on your needs, you may choose either a licensed practical nurse or a registered nurse. The former performs under the auspices of a physician and can give medications, develop a nursing-care plan, and document the individual's medical progress. Registered nurses can practice independently and do the same duties as a practical nurse, plus perform medical treatments and instruct you in nursing techniques.

Physical or Occupational Therapists

These professionals can help the individual with Alzheimer's cope with everyday skills, such as eating, bathing, and brushing teeth. They can also instruct you on proper transfer techniques, how to use shower chairs, and the correct installation of grab bars and handrails.

Social Workers

"When my husband was diagnosed with Alzheimer's, I didn't have any family nearby to turn to," said Molly. "I didn't know where to look for help, so my doctor gave me the number of the county office on aging. They connected me with a social worker, and she's been a godsend. She explained all the things I need to do—legal and financial matters, how to get home nursing, where I can join a support group."

Social workers can be an invaluable resource. They can put you in touch with community services such as meals, home health care, legal advice, and transportation. Many social workers offer counseling services for both you and the individual with Alzheimer's.

Social workers are affiliated with hospitals, public social service agencies (look in the Yellow Pages under "Social Services Organizations"), nursing homes, your local office of the state department of health, and some senior citizen centers. Many are also in private practice.

Other Health Professionals

Your pharmacist is an important member of the health care team, since he or she can help coordinate medications, inform you about potential side effects, and help prevent adverse drug interactions.

A dentist sensitive to the needs of people with Alzheimer's is another vital team member, especially when ill-fitting dentures prevent the person from speaking clearly or properly chewing food.

Occasionally the services of a nutritionist are needed if a person has special dietary needs or problem eating behaviors, such as refusing to eat many types of food. Your physician or social worker can make a recommendation.

A psychologist or psychiatrist can help individuals who are in the early stages of Alzheimer's cope with the realities of the disease and depression. Referrals for these professionals can come from your physician, although many caregivers prefer recommendations from other caregivers.

Some people may enlist the services of holistic practitioners to work in conjunction with medical specialists. These may include a person who administers biofeedback, a homeopathic or herbal practitioner, or a yoga, tai chi, or meditation teacher.

Other Professionals

Your caregiving responsibilities will be easier if, in addition to health care professionals, you also select experts in other fields to work with. These may include an attorney familiar with issues of elder law, a financial advisor, and a clergyman or other counselor to call upon in times of emotional stress.

As you make the many adjustments necessary to become a caregiver for the person with Alzheimer's, always bear in mind that the course of the illness is unique to the person. By the same token your caregiving experience will be unique, since you bring to the role skills, experiences, and a history with the person you're caring for that will affect all aspects of the process now and in the weeks, months, and years to come. Although it is helpful to read about and meet with other Alzheimer's caregivers, it is pointless to compare the illness of the person you're caring for with someone else's experience. Since the disease affects every person somewhat differently, it's best to focus on the needs of your own particular situation.

The following chapters will give you many specific techniques to help with the consequences of Alzheimer's disease, including problems with memory, communication, mood, behavior, movement, eating, exercise, and social activities. By implementing these strategies one day at a time you will help enrich the remaining years of the person you're caring for while taking the best possible care of yourself as well.

TWO

What You Need to Know About Alzheimer's Disease

"I just keep thinking, 'If only they had a cure, or some kind of treatment that could slow this thing down.' I read every article in the newspaper, every book—and they all say the same thing: We're hopeful about this, looking at that. But nothing is firm. They can do so many things now that could never be done before. Why can't they help people with Alzheimer's?"

—*Frank*

If you are like most people with a spouse, other family member, or close friend who has been diagnosed with Alzheimer's, you probably have many questions about the disease. In this chapter we'll answer the most commonly asked questions about Alzheimer's disease, including how a diagnosis is made, what the symptoms are, and what treatments are available to help alleviate symptoms.

WHAT IS ALZHEIMER'S DISEASE?

Alzheimer's disease is named after Alois Alzheimer, M.D., a German psychiatrist. In 1905 Dr. Alzheimer first described changes in the brain tissue of a woman who had died of an unknown mental illness. He found abnormal deposits (now called *senile* or *neuritic plaques*) and tangled bundles of nerve fibers (now known as *neurofibrillary tangles*) in the brain of his former patient. These plaques and tangles are characteristic abnormalities of the brain of a person with Alzheimer's.

WHAT CAUSES ALZHEIMER'S DISEASE?

The cause of the disease—the factors that cause buildup of plaques and tangles, and whether these plaques and tangles are responsible for the symptoms of Alzheimer's —is not known. However, several theories have been proposed. According to the Alzheimer's Disease Education and Referral (ADEAR) Center, it seems clear that Alzheimer's disease is not caused by hardening of the arteries. Nor is there any evidence that it is contagious. Although emotional upsets and stress may temporarily make symptoms worse, they don't cause the disease.

Some scientists believe Alzheimer's may result from a chronic infection or the effects of some toxic chemical in the environment; however, there is no firm evidence to support these theories. Others believe that overproduction of a substance called *amyloid,* which is found in neuritic plaques, causes the disease.

Recent studies have shown a relationship between genetic factors and Alzheimer's. Approximately 15 percent of people with Alzheimer's have a family history of the disease, occasionally with a dominant pattern of inheritance (in which children with one affected parent have a 50 percent chance of inheriting the disease). This type of

Alzheimer's disease, known as *familial disease*, offers the most clear-cut connection between genes and disease development.

However, a genetic risk factor is also likely in what is called *sporadic, late-onset* (occurring after age sixty-five) *disease*—the most common form. There is evidence that the presence of a gene that produces a protein called $APOE_4$ (apolipoprotein 4) increases the risk of developing Alzheimer's. However, it is likely that the presence of the gene alone is not sufficient to cause disease and that other factors and possibly other genes play a role as well.

Determining the cause of Alzheimer's is the first step in finding a cure. Until a cure is found, Alzheimer's is considered a terminal illness. Generally individuals do not die of Alzheimer's itself but of the complications that are associated with it, such as pneumonia, heart failure, and infections.

What This Means for You

Until the cause of the disease has been determined, a treatment or cure cannot be found. Although progress is being made and scientists are hopeful that effective treatments will be developed before the end of the decade, there is no way of knowing whether this will be the case and, even if so, whether any such treatment would affect the course of the disease in the person for whom you are now caring.

Therefore you should still start planning immediately for the future, finding out as much as you can about the financial status and wishes of the person with Alzheimer's now, when the person may still retain many of his or her mental and emotional faculties. Areas to consider include the individual's will, gaining power of attorney, setting up trusts, and learning what you can about Medicare, veterans' benefits, and insurance. Chapter 10 explores these issues in detail.

You might also start thinking about alternative living arrangements in the event they are required down the road.

"A woman in my Alzheimer's caregivers' support group asked me at what point I would consider putting my husband in a long-term-care facility," said Sheila. "Her husband had just been diagnosed with Alzheimer's; mine was diagnosed two years ago. I told her, 'I think when he no longer knows who I am, and when I'm physically unable to help him anymore.' But that's such a hard question. We've been married for nearly fifty years. I don't know whether I could send him somewhere else to live."

The kinds of services and facilities that are available for long-term care are covered in chapter 9.

HOW IS ALZHEIMER'S DISEASE DIAGNOSED?

At this time Alzheimer's disease cannot be definitively diagnosed in a living patient. The appearance of plaques and neurofibrillary tangles can be noted only by examining brain tissue, which is usually done as part of an autopsy. Therefore a probable diagnosis of Alzheimer's disease is generally made by a clinical examination based on a person's medical history, a physical exam, neuropsychological tests, and other tests of the person's mental ability.

A patient history includes a review of present and past medical problems as well as an examination of the person's ability to carry out activities of daily living, such as grooming, feeding oneself, going to work, and carrying out chores at home.

Family and friends are often asked to give feedback about the person who is being evaluated. Some of the questions may include the following: Is the person capable of concentrating on an activity? Can he or she make correct change when handling money? Write out checks? Balance a checkbook? Follow a recipe when cooking? Carry on a conversation clearly and logically?

Neuropsychological tests are done to examine motor functions, such as coordination and balance, and sensory abilities, including sensitivity to pain. Tests are also given to determine an individual's ability to remember numbers and objects and his or her orientation to time, place, and person (for example, "What date does Christmas fall on?" and "Where were you born?").

In a small number of cases Alzheimer's-like symptoms may be caused by other medical conditions, such as thyroid problems, brain tumors, blood vessel disease in the brain, pernicious anemia, or vitamin B_{12} deficiency, or depression. Some of these conditions are treatable. That's why an accurate diagnosis is so important.

Other tests that are used to determine whether the person has Alzheimer's or another disease, and to detect any other medical problems, include blood and urine tests and an examination of spinal fluid, which is done by taking a small sample of fluid from the spinal cord.

Brain imaging such as computerized tomography (CT)

scanning, magnetic resonance imaging (MRI), magnetic resonance spectroscopy (MRS), or positron emission tomography (PET) scanning may also be used to detect abnormalities in the brain.

What This Means for You

According to the Alzheimer's Association, experts accurately diagnose the disease in up to 90 percent of cases. If you are not convinced by one doctor's diagnosis, you may want to get a second opinion. In fact if your physician cannot make a probable diagnosis after the first round of tests, he or she may recommend retesting in six months to a year. This is not uncommon; although a delay in diagnosis is stressful for both you and the person being tested, Alzheimer's is such a serious disease that physicians try to be as accurate as possible in their diagnosis.

Nevertheless it is important to obtain an accurate diagnosis as soon as reasonably possible. Even a devastating diagnosis such as Alzheimer's brings an end to the stress of uncertainty and permits you to start taking necessary steps.

WHAT ARE THE SYMPTOMS OF ALZHEIMER'S DISEASE?

As noted in chapter 1, Alzheimer's disease eventually causes changes in personality and relationships, and takes a physical and emotional toll. The symptoms occur in stages, the length of which vary from person to person.

In the early stage, people experience minor symptoms that are often attributed to emotional upset, stress, or jokingly passed off as "old age." They may misplace things ("I just had my keys in my hand; now I can't find them") or have a fear of going out, preferring to stay home or in other familiar environments.

Gradually individuals with Alzheimer's become more forgetful, particularly about recent events ("What do you mean we visited my sister yesterday? I haven't seen her in weeks."). They may forget to turn off the stove after cooking or, at the other extreme, may recheck over and over to see whether the stove was turned off. Questions may be repeated, even after you've answered them several times.

As the disease progresses, memory loss increases and other changes, such as confusion, combativeness, and other mood and behavior problems, are likely to appear. These symptoms and how to handle them are discussed in detail in chapters 3 and 4.

In the middle stages judgment and decision-making abilities decline markedly. The person can no longer engage in complex activities such as balancing a checkbook, shopping for food or clothing, or traveling alone. It's not uncommon for people with Alzheimer's disease to deny or be unaware of the full extent of their limitations, which can be a source of deep frustration both for them and for their caregivers.

"Alex had always handled our finances," said Carol. "When I noticed two checks for the electric bill on the counter, I looked in the checkbook. It was a mess. There were checks missing, with no amounts written in. When I called the bank, I found out we were overdrawn. Alex

had made a mortgage payment that was thousands of dollars more than it was supposed to be. He has no idea what he did wrong, and I had been denying the problem, pretending to myself it didn't exist. The truth is, I was frightened. I didn't think I could learn how to handle money. But I realized then that I had no choice."

In the later stages physical problems emerge, including loss of coordination, lack of personal hygiene, and incontinence. These difficulties, and how to manage them, are covered in more detail in chapter 5. Some individuals may be unable to eat and swallow certain types of food effectively. Strategies for helping with eating and swallowing are discussed in chapter 7.

What This Means for You

The pace of your caregiving and the range of responsibilities you must take on will be determined by the course of the disease. In some cases, especially if the person deteriorates rapidly, you may be forced to take on more than you feel ready to handle. That's why it's so important to get as much information as you can at the outset and to build a support network for your emotional, medical, and legal/financial needs as soon as possible.

WHAT IS THE TREATMENT?

Although no known treatment will diminish or stop the progression of the disease, scientists are working on developing several treatment approaches, based on their findings of probable causes.

Since the late 1970s researchers have been testing various agents (physostigmine, cholinergic agonists, L-deprenyl, and tacrine, for example) in hopes of finding one or more that will improve cognition, slow progression, or cure the disease. Thus far none have been very promising.

However, physicians can often treat the secondary symptoms of Alzheimer's disease, such as depression, hallucinations, agitation, anxiety, and sleeplessness, by prescribing psychotropic drugs. Although these drugs may control the problem behaviors, many also have undesirable side effects, such as increasing memory loss and confusion, incontinence, and drowsiness.

Some people find that nondrug techniques, such as relaxation exercises, yoga, visualization, and meditation, can calm the person and thus reduce the severity of symptoms.

What This Means for You

At the current time, treatment for Alzheimer's disease does not come in a pill. It comes from you and others who are working to help the person with Alzheimer's be as comfortable and content as possible while maintaining dignity.

If the individual is treated for secondary symptoms, learn all you can about each drug, including potential side effects and interactions with other drugs. Don't hesitate to ask your physician or pharmacist questions about any medications the person is taking.

You may also want to participate in one of the numerous research studies involving investigational and experimental drugs that are ongoing around the country. In order to conduct this type of research, which is known as *clinical trials,* scientists need the support of individuals with Alzheimer's disease and their caregivers.

Be aware that participation in a research project has potential risks and offers no guarantee of improvement. Do not sign up for a study hoping for a miracle cure. In some cases drug treatment may cause symptoms to worsen; in other cases the drug may produce temporary improvements, such as slowing of memory loss.

"Al had the chance to be in a drug trial. When they told us his symptoms might worsen, we were hesitant. We finally decided to try the study. We figured if we said no, we'd definitely gain nothing. If we said yes, at least there was a chance some good would come of it. So far, the drug doesn't seem to be having much of an effect on Al's symptoms, but it's only been a few months. We'll see what happens over time."

To be eligible, people with Alzheimer's usually must be in the earlier stages of disease and in otherwise good health. They must have a full-time caregiver who can attend all the required sessions with them, and they cannot be taking any drug that may interfere with the experimental drug.

To help decide whether a person with Alzheimer's should consider participating in a research study, the following questions need to be answered:

• What are the researchers hoping to determine? Are their goals—for example, slowing memory loss or reducing mood and behavior problems—consistent with the individual's needs?

- What are the risks and side effects associated with the drug?
- What are the chances the individual will be given a placebo and not the drug itself?
- How long will he or she be required to participate? Be aware that some studies last up to five years.
- What part will you, the caregiver, have in the study? Will you be required to maintain a daily diary or fill out questionnaires? How often must you bring the individual in for testing and follow-up? Will you be required to travel long distances to meet these requirements?
- How much will the study cost you? Will your expenses be reimbursed?
- After meeting and talking with the researchers, are you comfortable with them? Did they answer your questions to your satisfaction? Did they or someone on the team explain the consent form to you?
- How and when will you be informed about the results of the study?

In addition to traveling, the person with Alzheimer's will likely meet more doctors and undergo many tests. Bear in mind that these factors may create additional stress; on the other hand having an opportunity to possibly reduce symptoms while enhancing knowledge about the disease may outweigh these inconveniences.

To learn more about clinical trials in your area, talk with your physician and contact your local Alzheimer's Association chapter.

The number of research studies into the cause of Alzheimer's disease has been growing steadily in the last few years. Several important theories are being investigated. Every discovery in the area of Alzheimer's research adds another piece to the complicated jigsaw puzzle of the disease. The results of this research may or may not directly impact people who have already been diagnosed with probable Alzheimer's. But they are likely to benefit your children and future generations.

Now that you have an idea of the "big picture" of Alzheimer's as it stands currently, it's time to learn about the symptoms of the disease in more detail as they pertain to you and the person for whom you are caring. Using the strategies suggested here to cope with specific changes can make life easier and more rewarding for both of you.

THREE

Helping with Memory and Communication Problems

"About three years after he was diagnosed with Alzheimer's, John's memory started getting really bad. By then we were used to the fact that we needed to do a schedule for each day, and place signs on the refrigerator, bathroom door, and other rooms to remind him of the activities we had planned and to help orient him at home. But then John started forgetting words; he couldn't tell us what he wanted to eat for dinner, or when he felt pain or discomfort. It was hard to guess what he wanted. Within months he couldn't read the signs and stopped recognizing the neighbors. My heart was breaking. I tried so hard to help him. We played word games, and used pictures to help him express himself. It worked for a time, and he smiled when he understood. Now, five years after he was diagnosed, I'm beginning to accept that we'll need to find other living arrangements for him, or get some kind of live-in help. I still love him, but I'm exhausted. I'll do anything I can to prolong our time together, as long as John still understands what's going on."

—Joanne

Everyone experiences some slowing of mental processes as he or she ages. For many people mild memory lapses begin around age fifty. By age seventy the ability to reason and speak often deteriorates slightly. For the four million Americans with Alzheimer's disease, however, memory loss is drastic and progressive. It is the most characteristic symptom of Alzheimer's, and one that affects many other aspects of the disease. As we'll see in this chapter, memory loss affects communication because the individual begins to forget words and eventually loses the ability to read and write. Memory loss also affects mood and behavior, as described in the next chapter, because the person may become increasingly frustrated, combative, and depressed as memory loss continues to impair the ability to think and function.

At this point there is no known medical treatment to slow the progressive memory loss that occurs from damage to the brain in Alzheimer's disease. However, many professionals believe that exercises designed to stimulate memory, such as memory enhancement and reality orientation, may help stave off deterioration somewhat. These exercises, as well as other aids to memory and communication, are described in this chapter. Since these strategies can be very demanding, because the exercises need to be repeated many times daily, it would be helpful for you to enlist the assistance of friends and relatives to work with the person at specific times of the day or week. This can give you a much-needed rest, as well as the comfort of knowing that the person is still being cared for.

MEMORY LOSS

Memory loss is the earliest and most characteristic symptom of Alzheimer's disease. *Short-term memory*—which refers to memories of events that occurred from several seconds to several days or weeks ago—is the first type of memory to be affected. An example is when the person forgets to turn off the stove after cooking or forgets that he or she has just had a visit from a friend or relative. *Long-term memory*—which generally refers to events that occurred months or years ago and is also involved in remembering how to perform basic tasks—is affected in the middle and later stages as the person's ability to function deteriorates progressively.

Memory loss affects every aspect of the lives of people with Alzheimer's—their ability to communicate, work, play, and care for themselves. In the final stages of the disease they usually do not recognize their spouse, family, or friends. They no longer remember how to feed themselves or how to use the toilet.

In the early stages of the disease some people realize they are losing their memory and try to hide this fact from others.

"Stan and I had our own hardware store for twenty years," said his brother, Rodney. "Stan was always sharp, knew the inventory like the back of his hand. I noticed he had double ordered some hammers. When I asked him why, he got angry and said I was mistaken. Then I noticed he was writing notes to remind himself to call certain people and order certain items—but he was writing the same note three or four times. He knew he had a problem and was trying to hide it, but he couldn't even remember writing the notes. This was probably my first clue that something was wrong. I talked to his wife, and she admitted that Stan would agree to pick up the

laundry or buy something for dinner, not do it, and deny that he had ever agreed to it."

In the early stages communication may also be affected. Many people with Alzheimer's can still carry on normal conversations and socialize, but occasionally they will forget ordinary, everyday words.

Karen noticed her husband was looking around the kitchen as if he had lost something. When she asked him what he wanted, he said "the yellow things." Because they had yellow dishes, she asked if that was what he wanted. He said no. "Are these things something you eat?" When he said yes, she asked, "You want grapefruit?" "No, they're long," he said. "Oh, you mean bananas!"

In the middle stages, as the disease progresses and dementia becomes more severe, many individuals have trouble understanding verbal or written instructions. Pictures may be used to help them remember where certain items are or how to find the bathroom or other specific parts of the home. For example, Abigail taped pictures of orange juice and fruit on the refrigerator and cookies and crackers on the cabinets so that her husband, Lawrence, could find these snacks. She took photographs of his shirts, pants, socks, and underwear and taped them to the closet doors and bureau drawers. "I wanted him to do as much as he could for himself for as long as possible," she said.

In the later stages of Alzheimer's most memory is gone. People with Alzheimer's eventually cannot recognize anyone. Most if not all of their basic needs must be met for them by others.

COPING WITH MEMORY LOSS

Memory Aids

During the early stages numerous memory aids can be used to help people with Alzheimer's function as independently and safely as possible. The following strategies can be effective for individuals who have mild or moderate memory impairment:

- Write out instructions for performing tasks. A person with Alzheimer's may have done the laundry hundreds of times in the past, but now you cannot assume he or she will remember to turn on the water or add the soap. Notes to remind the person to "Wash Hands" or "Flush" can also be helpful.
- Place labels on the outside of cabinets, drawers, closet doors, and boxes to identify the contents. This will help the person with Alzheimer's find items he or she uses or needs frequently, such as clothing, books, photos, important papers, toiletry items, and kitchen utensils.
- Keep the surroundings uncluttered and don't shift furniture or other items from place to place. People with Alzheimer's function more easily in settings that are orderly and distraction-free. Moving furniture, television, radio, or even pictures on the wall may add to their confusion.
- Develop a daily routine, write it down, and post it. This does not mean you must account for every minute

of the day, but give the person with Alzheimer's a general idea of what will be happening. A daily schedule might be structured as follows: Shower, Get dressed, Breakfast, Garden, Lunch, Walk, Call friends, Prepare dinner, Read, Watch TV, Bedtime.

- Keep a large wall calendar visible and mark off each day. Write in upcoming activities (doctors' appointments, visits to or from others, shopping trips) and the time they will occur. Have at least one clock the individual can see easily. These strategies help people with Alzheimer's remember the day and time, and stay oriented in the here and now.

Memory-Enhancement Training

Some health care professionals believe individuals with mild to moderate levels of memory impairment can benefit from memory-enhancement programs. These techniques may slow the decline in memory and thus allow the person more time to do things he or she wants to do and to plan for the future. Whether such techniques truly help is open to question. Nevertheless if they can be performed with a minimum of inconvenience, they cannot hurt and can give the feeling of spending time constructively.

Memory-enhancement training involves the use of the memory aids described above, such as lists, calendars, and daily schedules. In addition other techniques are employed. For example the person with Alzheimer's is encouraged to pay attention to what he or she is doing and verbalize it to reduce absentminded behavior; when he or she places the keys to the house on the kitchen table, the person should say, "I am placing the keys on the kitchen table." Contact your local chapter of the Alzheimer's Association for more information on these programs.

Reality Orientation

Over time individuals with Alzheimer's disease may withdraw from contact with others and the environment as they become increasingly disoriented. This withdrawal results in a lack of sensory stimulation. To prevent understimulation, a therapy called *reality orientation* was developed. It is based on the belief that continually and repeatedly telling or showing certain reminders to people with mild to moderate memory loss will result in an increase in interaction with others and improved orientation. This in turn can improve self-esteem and reduce problem behaviors.

Reality orientation can be taught to caregivers and family members by a psychotherapist or other health care provider trained in these techniques. It can be performed in the home and should be structured around the area in which the person with Alzheimer's spends most of his or her time. Access to a window is recommended to facilitate orientation to the time of day and the weather.

In reality orientation, people with Alzheimer's are surrounded by familiar objects that can be used to stimulate their memory. Other materials, such as family scrapbooks, flash cards, Scrabble games, a globe, large-piece jigsaw puzzles, and illustrated, large-print dictionaries, are also used.

Another tool, the reality-orientation board, is any board with a surface on which information can be changed easily, such as a blackboard, a pegboard, or an erasable memo board. Both the caregiver and the person with Alzheimer's fill in information such as current day of the week, date, and year, and the weather.

When Myrna's mother came to live with Myrna and her family, Myrna followed the therapist's advice for preparing her living space. "We put up a large clock, a wall calendar, and a bulletin board where we could post her hourly activities. We also bought a television and a radio for her room, and displayed framed photographs of family members and friends. Mom has a thimble collection, and we put that on her wall." The therapist advised Myrna to hold daily discussions with her mother about family members, television shows, movies, recipes, and current events. Every day her mother spent some time looking at the daily newspaper and current magazines.

Reality orientation can also be used for persons who are more severely confused. For these individuals, however, work focuses on less complicated information, such as their own name and address, the name of their caregiver, colors, and identification of everyday objects.

Reality orientation is around-the-clock therapy; the caregiver and anyone who has contact with the person with Alzheimer's should be encouraged to apply the techniques. General guidelines include the following:

- Treat people with memory impairment with respect. Do not talk down to them or treat them like children.
- Every conversation you have with the person should include mention of the time of day, day of the week, and names of familiar people and objects.
- People with Alzheimer's should be encouraged to perform activities of daily living—that is, getting dressed,

eating, taking care of personal hygiene—and should be complimented on all such attempts.

• When individuals have confused or mistaken beliefs about people, things, or time, their notions should be corrected—that is, brought back to reality—tactfully and lovingly. For example, despite the obvious sunshine streaming through the window, Eric said it was raining. Martha took him gently by the arm and led him to the window. "The rain is gone, Eric," she said. "The sun is shining now. Can you feel the warm sun on your face?"

Reminiscence Technique

Although short-term memory fades during the mild and moderate stages of the disease, long-term memory remains. Some caregivers put this fact to use by encouraging individuals to talk about the past. This technique was developed in the 1960s by Dr. Robert Butler, who called it *life review*.

The reminiscence technique can be used by anyone willing to listen to a person with Alzheimer's who is willing to talk. Caregivers, and especially the grandchildren of individuals with Alzheimer's disease, are good candidates as listeners.

Advocates of the technique say that reminiscence builds self-esteem because it allows people with Alzheimer's to focus on things they can remember rather than be frustrated by what they cannot remember. Some believe that calling upon long-term memory stimulates memory function in general and may help a person's mind remain active for a longer time. "My twelve-year-old daughter and ten-year-old son sit with their grandfather once a week and ask him questions about his child-

HELPING WITH MEMORY AND COMMUNICATION PROBLEMS | 39

hood, life on the farm, what he did in school, places he visited—he never seems to run out of memories," said Vera. "It has a very calming effect on him—so much so that on other occasions when I see him becoming agitated, I get him to talk about 'the good old days.'"

Suggestions for using the reminiscence technique include the following:

- Ask specific questions about the past that require more than a yes-or-no answer. Instead of "Did you like going to school?" ask "What kinds of things did you learn in grade school?"
- Pose follow-up questions to help the person continue his or her narration, such as "Was that a hard job?" or "How were you able to do that?"
- Encourage the individual to talk about his or her past achievements, talents, or skills: "I heard you used to be quite a dancer"; "Your apple pies were legendary in town"; "How did your flower shop outsell all the others in town?"
- Acknowledge and validate the person's feelings, both positive and negative. "It sounds like you had a wonderful time that day." "It was wrong of them to cheat you on that deal. I would be angry too."
- Remember that your job is to listen; keep your comments brief, and don't interrupt the speaker.
- Some memories may be painful. If the speaker looks or acts upset or uncomfortable, change the subject.
- Use sensory cues—old photographs, the smell of hot apple pie, foods he or she used to eat, old songs or music, the feel of a velvet dress—to assist in recall. "Before my husband and I were married, we used to go to the drugstore every Friday to have a chocolate malt," said Al-

lison. "Well, we hadn't had a malt since then. So I made two chocolate malts, and when I put one down in front of Ray, you should have seen the smile on his face. That malt started a flood of memories."

- Prompt the person by recalling specific events or dates in the past, such as their eighteenth birthday, the day they got their first car, their first job, their first kiss.

Reminiscence sessions can be therapeutic for the person with Alzheimer's disease and informative for you and other listeners. They are an excellent way for family members with Alzheimer's to participate in family gatherings.

MEMORY-RELATED COMMUNICATION PROBLEMS

Phil wanted a pizza, but the only words he could say to convey it were "hot" and "round." This is typical of one type of memory-related communication problem experienced by people with Alzheimer's—difficulty finding the right words to express themselves to others. On the other hand, some individuals have trouble understanding what people are saying to them, or immediately forget what they've just heard.

When the Person Can't Express Himself

When people with Alzheimer's have trouble finding the right words to communicate their thoughts, they may describe an item they cannot name, or substitute words that have a similar sound or meaning.

"Larry, I want the music thing."
"Do you mean the radio, Catherine?"
"No, it sings songs."
"Can you tell me what it looks like?"
"It's like a hula hoop." This made him stop for a minute. Did she mean it was round?
"Do you mean a record?"
"Yes, that's it."

Larry made the connection rather quickly and without his wife becoming upset because he remained calm and did not pressure her. It takes much patience to communicate with individuals who forget names, struggle for the words they want to use, never finish a sentence, or repeat the same phrase over and over—all problems that may be experienced by people with Alzheimer's disease. To facilitate communication, try these strategies:

- Relax. People with Alzheimer's communicate better when they do not feel pressured.
- Keep distractions to a minimum. Turn off the radio and television. If other people are in the room, find a quiet spot.
- When the person has trouble expressing a thought, guess what may be meant by asking questions they can answer with a yes or no. For example, "Do you mean . . . ?" or "Do you want to go to . . . ?"
- Sometimes people forget what they were saying and stop in the middle of a sentence. To help them start again, calmly repeat the last few words they said. If they can't continue, ask a question that relates to what they had been saying.
- Make sure you understand what they have said.

Questions like "You want to leave now, is that right?" or "You want some milk, don't you?" will verify what's been said.

- You may have to decipher a meaning from a few words. The person's tone of voice and body language may also help you figure out what they mean. For example, a shaky voice and fidgeting behavior may convey fear more than their words can. Many people have limited access to the words they want to use. "Walk now" may mean a person is uncomfortable and wants to leave the room.

When the Person Can't Understand You

People with memory loss may understand what you tell them but then quickly forget what they understood. Francine noticed this problem with her husband. "I told Bradley, 'I'm going to work in the garden. I'll be back in thirty minutes. Do you understand?' He said he understood, but then a few minutes later he started yelling for me. He had already forgotten where I was."

Jeff said "I asked my dad, 'Would you like soup for lunch?' and he said yes. Then when I gave it to him, he said no." So Jeff asked his father if he wanted flowers for dinner. When his father answered yes again, Jeff realized that even though his father answered his questions in the affirmative, he didn't really understand what his son was asking. Now Jeff backs up his questions about food choices by showing his father a picture or the actual item.

You can help keep the communication lines open between you and individuals with Alzheimer's by using such reinforcements. In addition, try the following strategies:

- If the person wears a hearing aid or glasses, be sure they are the correct prescription and are working properly.
- Keep background music and other distractions to a minimum.
- To get the person's attention and help maintain his or her concentration, frequently address the person by name, maintain eye contact, and gently touch his or her hand or arm.
- Speak clearly and slowly, using simple words and phrases. "Bill, please give me the book" is more likely to be understood than "Bill, I want you to pick up that book and hand it to me."
- Be specific about things, places, and activities. Say "Let's go to the store" rather than "Let's go out"; "Do you want an apple?" rather than "Do you want some fruit?"
- When you need to repeat a statement or question, use the same words each time. If "Betty, please give me the pillow" does not prompt Betty to get the pillow, repeat the request exactly the same way. "Toss the pillow over here" will only confuse the person.
- Use flash cards. Simple drawings or photographs pasted on cardboard can help you communicate, especially with individuals who have lost most or all of their verbal skills. Use pictures of a toilet, bathtub, lamp, items of clothing, pillow, blanket, bed, toothbrush, glasses, and food items.
- Act out an activity you want performed. Actions like eating, drinking, walking, sitting, lying down, and comb-

ing hair are easy to show. "Beverly has forgotten how to brush her teeth," said William. "I put toothpaste on her brush and on mine, put the brush in her hand, hold it up to her mouth, and then I brush my teeth. She mimics me, although sometimes I have to coax her."

Using such strategies becomes an integral part of day-to-day living and caring for a person with Alzheimer's disease. It can be a frustrating and disheartening experience for the caregiver, especially when the person is a loved one whose capabilities were relied upon and respected. Nevertheless for many people the reward of maintaining contact and possibly slowing the course of the disease are well worth the effort.

In the next chapter we'll look at how Alzheimer's disease affects the person's mood and behavior, and suggest strategies for coping with potential problems as well as limiting their severity.

FOUR

Helping with Mood and Behavior Problems

"The first thing I noticed was that Margaret started pacing a lot. She couldn't seem to sit still, not even in the evening, when we had always enjoyed sitting and watching television after dinner. Then she started mumbling to herself, and talking to her aunt, Isabelle, a woman who passed away ten years ago! It did no good to tell Margaret that Aunt Isabelle wasn't around anymore; she insisted I was wrong. Then one night, when I was preparing dinner, she started screaming that I was trying to poison her! I was devastated! My wife of forty years thought I was trying to kill her. I felt frightened, disoriented. I was living with a madwoman! I called my daughter, who rushed over. She calmed Margaret down by singing lullabies. But she couldn't calm me down. I didn't know what to do, how to feel. My daughter insisted I tell the doctor, who prescribed some medication. But I'm frightened, very frightened by Margaret's behavior. Who would ever believe this would happen?"

—Morris

Mood and behavior problems are among the earliest symptoms in people with Alzheimer's disease. The consequences can be devastating to caregivers, who may find themselves living with a person they no longer recognize.

In this chapter we'll examine these problems, which may include anxiety and nervousness, wandering, combativeness, violent behavior, clinging, depression, hallucinations, delusions, and hoarding (of food or other items). Changes in sexual behavior will also be covered.

It's important to remind yourself that the person with Alzheimer's often has little control over his or her emotions and actions. Some caregivers find it difficult to accept that the person is not trying to inflict harm or damage intentionally. "When my mother curses and tries to hit me, I know she doesn't know what she's doing," said Bert. "I see fear in her eyes. She doesn't even know who I am sometimes. I have to keep telling myself that somewhere in there is the gentle, soft-spoken mother I once knew."

Although the mood and behavior problems experienced by people with Alzheimer's are caused by damage to the brain, there are still steps you can take to reduce or limit their severity, especially in the early and middle stages of the disease. We will present strategies that many caregivers have found to be effective in curbing some of these destructive symptoms.

ANXIETY AND NERVOUSNESS

Although anxiety and nervousness may result from changes in chemicals in the brain, they may also occur when the person with Alzheimer's experiences feelings of loss, confusion, or fear. For example, anxiety is common in the early stages of the illness when individuals realize they are losing their ability to function and are not thinking or behaving as they did formerly.

"I'm all messed up. I can't do anything right anymore." Betty, who was recently diagnosed with probable Alzheimer's disease, constantly voices these concerns to her husband, Leonard. He noted that Betty also keeps saying that he will leave her. *"I reassure her all the time that I love her and won't leave, but it doesn't seem to help much. In fact her constant fear is driving me away. I keep having to remind myself that it's not Betty's fault that she's behaving this way. But it's hard. I never had to talk this way to her before; she was always so confident. Now I have to be the strong one."*

As the disease progresses, some people with Alzheimer's also become anxious and nervous when in an unfamiliar setting, such as a store or doctor's office. Or, for no apparent reason, they may begin worrying about people who have died ("Where's my mother? Why doesn't my father call me?"). Anxiety over the loss of a particular item or about a specific event is also common. For example they may insist they have lost their car or a ring they sold long ago.

"Sometimes my mother doesn't recognize my father and keeps looking around the house for him," said Louise. *"She goes from room to room, looking in closets and under tables, saying, 'Ollie, where are you? I know you're here.' She walks up to him and orders him to help her find Ollie! He goes along with her. It does no good to tell her that he's here. At first my father was astounded; he thought she was playing games with him. Now he just accepts it as part of the disease. But it's weird for anyone else who happens to be there with them."*

Fidgeting, restlessness, irritability, and pacing are also symptoms of anxiety and nervousness. "My husband turns on all the faucets and then turns them off," said Edith. "Then he pulls the books off the shelves and puts them back. I'm glad he at least puts them back! But that behavior makes *me* anxious."

It is important to try to alleviate the person's feelings of anxiety and nervousness, since they may lead not only to problem behaviors but also to injuries, especially if the person insists upon doing an activity that is potentially dangerous. "My wife was very restless, so I gave her laundry to fold," said Irv. "That satisfied her for a while, but then she wanted to iron. She irons everything over and over again. I have to watch her constantly. One day I walked out of the room for just a few seconds and she left the iron on a shirt and scorched it. Fortunately it didn't start a fire."

To help relieve feelings of anxiety and nervousness, try:

• Giving verbal and nonverbal reassurances—"I'm glad we're together today"—coupled with a hug or holding the person's hand can be comforting, especially if you see he or she is frustrated during activities such as eating or dressing. Speak in a calm, relaxed tone and make eye contact.

• Scheduling chores such as folding laundry, raking leaves, or dusting during the day to provide activities and to structure time.

• Keeping instructions for an activity simple. Do not pressure the person to rush through a task.

• Encouraging physical activity, such as a walk, gardening, or playing catch. For example Edith's husband enjoyed hitting a tennis ball against the outside garage wall. This kept him busy, and she could keep an eye on him when she hung up the laundry.

- Playing music. "My sister is much less anxious when I play big-band music. I even bought a cassette to play in the car. When I'm tired of listening to it, I give her my portable cassette player and earphones, and she walks around the house swaying to Benny Goodman!"
- Eliminating caffeine products, such as coffee, tea, chocolate, and cola, from the diet. Many people experience agitation and anxiety after ingesting these products.
- Avoiding difficult or stressful activities when the person is tired and less able to sustain concentration.

WANDERING AND RESTLESSNESS

"A few months ago Bonnie started to wander around the house as if she were looking for something," said Tom. "She goes in and out of all the rooms. After about twenty minutes she stops. Sometimes she does this three or four times a day." Tom became alarmed when he left the room for a few minutes one day and found Bonnie gone when he returned. She had walked out the front door and was about to step into the street when Tom grabbed her.

"She said she was going to see our daughter. Our daughter lives in Canada, and we live in Florida. I was afraid for her safety, but I didn't want to lock her inside our house. A friend suggested I hang a bell over all the outside doors so that I can hear when she tries to leave the house."

Needless to say, wandering can be a dangerous problem. Some people take the car and drive until they become lost or have an accident. Chronic wanderers may need constant supervision. Those who become lost or disoriented may be frightened and hide, making it difficult to find them.

Wandering may be in response to a specific event, such as starting to attend a new day-care center or moving into the home of a relative. Some believe wandering activity may be an attempt to find something familiar in these new surroundings. Boredom, restlessness, or a need for more exercise may also trigger wandering behavior.

Some individuals with Alzheimer's appear to wander for no reason. For example Eric gets up every morning at six o'clock and wanders around the house and yard for more than an hour. His wife, Martha, has to get up and make sure he doesn't hurt himself.

"I have no idea why he does it," Martha said. "When I ask him, he never answers me. Of course it bothers me, mostly because I'm afraid one day I won't get up in time and he'll have an accident. With this disease you're always on guard for something."

Wandering behavior can be dangerous if the environment is unsafe. To help prevent accidents:

- Keep sharp objects, matches, toxic cleaning supplies, and medicines out of sight and out of reach.
- Remove the knobs on the stove and keep them out of reach.
- Install room monitors so that you can hear what the person is doing in another room.
- Place a security gate across stairs. Lock doors and windows.

- Install childproof doorknob covers or spring-operated latches, which are difficult for people with Alzheimer's to use.
- Hang bells on all the doors that lead outside so that you can hear when the person tries to leave.
- Ask your neighbors to call you if they see the individual out alone.

Some people with Alzheimer's are obviously agitated when they wander. "My father stomps around the house mumbling," said Troy. "He marches up the stairs to the bedroom, stomps around, then goes to the living room and does the same thing. He has a very determined look on his face, and if you try to talk to him, he waves his arms and tries to hit you. He does this for hours without stopping. It can be kind of frightening."

Reactions to medications such as tranquilizers or antidepressants cause some people to become restless and confused (see chapter 6), thereby triggering wandering behavior. Discuss this possibility with your physician.

Other strategies for coping with wandering include the following:

- Anticipate and plan for wandering when possible. Any change in environment or living arrangements is less likely to cause wandering if it is made early in the course of the illness when the individual might understand why the move is being made. If possible, include the person in the decision-making process. For example when Robert and his wife realized his mother, Beatrice, would eventually need constant care, they made arrangements for her to move from her apartment in New York to their home in Philadelphia. Before she moved in permanently, Beatrice visited her son's family several times so that her new surroundings would feel more familiar when she made the final move.

The same is true if you are considering enrolling the person in a day-care center. People with Alzheimer's are less likely to wander if they begin going to the center early in their illness. Keep the first few visits short, and stay with the person.

If possible, have a representative from the center visit the person with Alzheimer's at home before he or she begins to attend the facility on a regular basis. This will help the person feel more comfortable and safe once the transition is made.

- Distract the wanderer by offering a favorite food or beverage, or suggesting an activity. Carl uses several techniques to keep his wife, Priscilla, from wandering in the yard. "First, I ask her to help me do something, such as going through our photo collection," he said. "If that doesn't work, I tell her we're going to make cookies or tea. When all else fails, I walk with her and try to lead her back to the house."

- Look for patterns in the wandering behavior. Does the person always wander at the same time of day or after doing a certain activity? If so, you can distract the individual before he or she tries to wander. If certain items trigger the desire to wander, such as keys, an overcoat, or a briefcase, put these items out of sight.

- Some people wander because they need more physical activity. Involve the individual in more chores. Add a daily, vigorous walk to the routine. If the person tends to wander at night, take a long walk with him or her late in the day.

- Wandering may be an indication that the person

needs to attend to a basic need, such as going to the bathroom or having a drink of water. For example several months after Paul moved in with his daughter, Desiree, he began wandering around the house. "He couldn't remember where the bathroom was," Desiree said. "I didn't realize that although he had no trouble finding it when he first moved in with me, now his memory was worse." She taped a "Bathroom" sign with an arrow in the hallway and another on the bathroom door to help him.

- Reassure the person with Alzheimer's that he or she is safe and wanted. Daily reminders that you are glad to be with the person may lessen the urge to wander.
- Permit a certain amount of wandering if necessary. Individuals who are agitated while wandering may be difficult to handle. Attempts to stop them may only make them more disturbed or confused.

Regardless of why people with Alzheimer's wander, it's a good idea to purchase an ID bracelet for them. You can buy one from a jewelry store or purchase a "Medic Alert" bracelet from a pharmacy. The ID should be engraved with "Alzheimer's/Memory-impaired" and a telephone number to call when the person is found. An identification card carried in the person's wallet or pocket is an alternative, but cards are more likely to be lost than a bracelet.

An excellent way to protect wanderers is through a service called the Helmsley Alzheimer's Alert Program, which maintains a twenty-four-hour hot line and service that will help the caregiver find a lost Alzheimer's patient. When the person enrolls (at no charge), he or she receives a bracelet engraved with his or her ID number and the toll-free hot-line number. Contact your local Alzheimer's Association office for more information.

COMBATIVENESS AND ANGER

People with Alzheimer's may, without warning or apparent provocation, become irate and abusive, verbally and physically. They may throw objects, scream, kick, bite, or strike out at their caregiver or others. Because people with Alzheimer's cannot explain these outbursts, researchers are uncertain about what causes them. They may reflect the person's unconscious fears or anger, or they may be caused by brain damage.

"Every time I try to wash my mother's hair, she screams and tries to hit me," said Mary. "She allows me to help her bathe, but she won't get her head wet. We took her to my cousin's beauty shop after hours, but she threw the shampoo bottles at us. The best we can do is use a dry shampoo."

These violent episodes can be justifiably frightening and upsetting to caregivers and other family members and friends. The first step in attempting to reduce the frequency or severity of such behavior is to identify potential triggers. One such trigger for many people with Alzheimer's is fear of water. As you will see in chapter 5, it can be helpful to use a shower chair and handheld shower hose to bathe the person from the feet up, rather than having water run down on his or her head.

Other triggers of combative behavior may include:

- A task with many steps, which can be confusing and frustrating. For example, getting dressed may be overwhelming for some individuals unless you turn it into a structured, step-by-step experience (see chapter 5).
- Trying to rush the person or acting upset.
- Not understanding what you are telling her or asking her to do. Feelings of frustration may lead to combativeness.
- Not being able to make himself understood. For example, Phil becomes very abusive when his wife, Arlene, doesn't understand what he wants to eat. "The other day he said 'round' and I asked 'apple'? Then he shouted, 'Round, hot.' When I showed him a can of tomato soup, he grabbed it and threw it on the floor. The 'round, hot' he wanted was pizza. He calmed down when I took a pizza out of the freezer."
- Noisy, crowded, or unfamiliar surroundings, such as a restaurant or family gathering.
- Illness or fatigue. Frustration increases in most people when they are in pain or have not had adequate sleep.

In addition to identifying triggers, there are other steps you can take to limit combativeness. These may include the following:

- At the first sign of frustration, remain calm. For example, John's father started cursing when trying to put on his shirt. John patted him on the back and said, "It's okay. Take your time. There's no rush."
- Keep your explanations and instructions simple. Use short, simple sentences, such as "Let's go into the living room. I'll put on the television." Also use encouraging phrases such as "that's good" and "you're doing fine."

- Maintain eye contact with the person as much as possible. This can give you a feeling of being in charge and in control, which is then conveyed to the person you're caring for.

- Distract the person from a task that is causing anxiety. When John's father had trouble buttering a piece of bread, John suggested he eat the mashed potatoes first and return to the bread later.

- Determine which activities are soothing to the person. Donna discovered that her husband forgets his anger when they dance. "I put a tape into the recorder and start to dance by myself," she says. "Then I ask Neil to join me. I learned that I can't grab his arm first; he has to come to me on his own. Most of the time it works. We dance for a few minutes and then he forgets why he was upset." Other things that may calm a person include holding a stuffed animal, stroking a pet, or watching fish in an aquarium.

- If the person seems receptive, pat her hand, hug her, or slowly rock her. Some people may not want to be touched, however, or they may experience rocking as a form of restraint. Use your own judgment.

- Keep a record of outbursts and look for a pattern. Note what happens, who was there, when it happened and where, and what happened just before the person became aggressive. Did the individual seem restless in the moments preceding the incident? Overly tired? Was there a lot of confusion or noise in the environment? Was he or she upset when a particular person came into the room?

Sometimes despite your best efforts the person with Alzheimer's may become so violent that he is a danger to himself or to you. If you find yourself in a potentially

HELPING WITH MOOD AND BEHAVIOR PROBLEMS | 57

dangerous situation, take the following steps to protect yourself and the person in your care:

- Do not attempt to restrain or hold the individual. You may end up hurting yourself and the person unnecessarily.
- Step back five or six steps from the person and remain quiet. Wait to see if he or she calms down alone. Many people with Alzheimer's who are hostile become manageable after a few minutes. "Lila picked up a brass candlestick and swung it at me," said her husband. "Then she just stood there and shouted, 'I hate you.' I picked up a pillow, held it in front of me, and started singing 'The Yellow Rose of Texas,' her favorite song, real low. After a minute she started to cry. I wanted to put my arms around her, but I just kept singing until she stopped crying. Then I felt safe."
- Protect yourself with an object you can use as a shield—a pillow, chair, box, wastebasket.
- Use your shield to maneuver the person into a corner, preferably away from doors or windows that the individual could use to escape and possibly hurt himself or herself.
- Do not shout or scream. Either remain silent or talk in a low monotone. People with Alzheimer's tend to imitate what they see and sense. If you remain calm, they may become calm too.
- If the person grabs you, go limp. Do not fight back.
- Call friends, relatives, or neighbors for help as soon as possible. If you believe your safety or that of the individual is in jeopardy, call 911 or the local medical emergency number. Medical personnel are more likely to be

trained to handle a person who has Alzheimer's disease than are the police.

If aggression and combativeness become a problem, as they frequently do as the disease progresses, your physician may prescribe tranquilizers, such as diphenhydramine, thioridazine, haloperidol, or oxazepam. Side effects of these drugs are described in chapter 6. Physical restraints are usually avoided unless the individual has injured someone.

CLINGING BEHAVIOR

"It's like the song 'Me and My Shadow,'" Polly said. "Bill follows me everywhere, even into the bathroom. I guess he thinks he'll lose me if he lets me out of his sight."

Clinging behavior is one way some individuals with Alzheimer's seek a feeling of security in their very confused lives. They identify the caregiver as the one person they can depend on; he or she is their tenuous link with the world. Clinging is a way of not losing you or feeling abandoned. The person with Alzheimer's may forget, for example, that when you go to work in the morning, you will return in the afternoon, or that you will reemerge from the bathroom after several minutes.

Being followed all the time can be very stressful. Here are strategies you can use to help you cope with this annoying behavior and create space for yourself:

- Give the person a task or chore he or she can do unsupervised for ten or twenty minutes. When Claire wants time to take a shower, she gives her sister, Paula, some clothes to fold. "Even if I don't have anything for her to fold, I unload a few drawers. It keeps her busy for about twenty minutes." Other tasks include dusting, sorting socks or buttons, or stacking books and magazines.
- Ask a relative or friend to stay with the individual while you take a nap or go out.
- To reassure the person with Alzheimer's that you will come back from your outing, draw a picture of a clock showing the time you will return. Place it near a real clock and tell them you'll be back when the two clocks are alike.
- For short breaks at home set an alarm clock or oven timer and tell the individual you will be back when the bell rings.
- Give the person headphones to listen to soft music. Tapes of his or her favorite music may have a calming effect.

DEPRESSION

Depression appears to be more common in the early stages of the illness, when individuals realize they are losing their memory and other abilities. About 25 percent of individuals with Alzheimer's are depressed. Restlessness, suicidal thoughts, feelings of hopelessness, difficulty concentrating, and withdrawing are signs of depression. Getting up at two or four o'clock in the morning complaining of anxiety and being unable to go back to sleep is another common sign.

Psychotherapy or another form of group or individual counseling can help men and women who still have most of their memory learn to accept their progressive memory loss and how to compensate for it. Other strategies for alleviating depression include the following:

- Keeping the lines of communication open. Let the person know you are available to listen if he wants to talk about his feelings.
- Avoiding giving the person "pep talks" or false hopes. It's better to deal as calmly and compassionately as possible with the reality of the situation.
- Encouraging exercise and social interaction. People who feel uncomfortable being in crowds or socializing, however, should not be forced to participate. Having friends or relatives visit on a one-to-one basis is an alternative. Yoga exercises, which can be particularly calming, can be done at home.
- Encouraging the use of meditation, visualization, and related activities that calm the mind and body.
- Discouraging the use of alcohol, which, after an initial feeling of euphoria, can actually increase feelings of depression.

Although antidepressants are an option, many physicians prefer not to prescribe these drugs because of the potential side effects, which may include tremor, confusion, anxiety, and cardiac effects. However, when drugs are indicated, amitriptyline, doxepin, nortriptyline, desipramine, and fluoxetine are commonly prescribed. See chapter 6 for more information.

HALLUCINATIONS

Hallucinations are perceptions of things, smells, sounds, physical sensations, or tastes that are not truly there. People may hear voices when no one is around; they may smell a roast when nothing is cooking. Some hallucinations are terrifying to people with Alzheimer's disease and can cause them to become agitated or afraid to go to sleep. "Sometimes Cliff insists there are planes circling the bed," said Rhoda. "He yells, 'they're diving, they're diving' and then covers his head with the sheet. Other times he tells me the room is full of birds. When I ask him what kind, he describes them to me. They're very frightening to him and to me."

If the person you're caring for experiences hallucinations, the first thing to do is to schedule a physical examination. Treatable conditions that may cause hallucinations include drug or alcohol abuse, dehydration, bladder or kidney infections, and intense pain.

Try the following strategies when hallucinations occur:

- Remain calm. Don't tell the person, "You're crazy," or "You don't really see that."
- Gently reassure the person that you are there to help. Offer to hold his or her hand. Say "I'm here to protect you," or "I'll stay here with you. Don't worry."
- Distract the individual by suggesting you both go for a walk or get something to eat. Washing the person's face with cold water can also dispel hallucinations.
- Be honest. "Should I agree with Miranda when she says she hears bees buzzing through the house?" asked Wayne. "She keeps asking me, 'Do you hear them? Can't you hear them?' What should I say?" Acknowledge that

the hallucination is real for her, but that you do not hear or see what she does. Now Wayne tells his wife, "I know you hear bees in the house, but I don't hear them."

- Be aware that in some cases the hallucination is merely an exaggeration of something grounded in reality. As children we all saw the "boogey man" lurking in our bedroom shadows, but when the light went on, no one was there. Shadows, dark hallways, glare from lights or the sun, fog, and even items around the house may look threatening to a person with Alzheimer's disease. "My wife began to cry and said she was going to be sucked into the dark cave," said Ron. "As I hugged her and told her I would protect her, I realized I had left the dryer door open. From across the room it looked like a dark hole. When I moved toward it, she got hysterical. I shut the door and reassured her that the cave was gone and we were safe."

If these strategies are not effective, your physician may prescribe medication (see chapter 6).

DELUSIONS

A delusion is a belief system that has no basis in reality. For example, the person you are caring for may think he or she is Jesus or Eleanor Roosevelt. "Wanda tells me she is the queen and that her knights are coming to visit her," said Ray. "She asks me, 'Can you see their horses yet?' and I answer, 'No, I don't see anything. Please help me set the table.' Or I suggest we take a walk."

Calling the person's attention to the immediate surroundings—offering food, asking how he likes the weather—seems to be the most effective way of bringing him out of an episode of delusion; however, it won't always work. The most you can do is to accept the fact that you can't change the person's thoughts. No amount of reasoning will convince Wanda she is not the queen. As long the delusions are harmless, as many of them are, all you can hope to do is make the person comfortable, safe, and reasonably happy.

PARANOIA

Closely related to delusions are feelings of paranoia and suspicion. When people can't remember where they put their money or other possessions, they may accuse others of stealing them. "My aunt has diamond necklaces and rings, which we put in a safe-deposit box," said Mollie. "When she asked to see them one day, my husband went to the bank and took them out of the box. By the time he got back, she had decided we were thieves. We showed her the jewelry, but she said it wasn't hers, that my husband had had counterfeit jewelry made and that we had taken hers."

Frequently the delusions of people with Alzheimer's are turned against their caregivers or family members. This can cause sadness and pain for the targets of the accusations. For example Herb believes his son is trying to kill him. Now Harry no longer can visit his father, and his mother can't let her husband know when she sees Harry. "Harry is very sad about his father," said Sarah. "I can't mention Harry's name in the house because Herb accuses me of being an accomplice."

To cope with paranoid behavior, try the following strategies:

- Never tell people with Alzheimer's they are "acting paranoid." If they believe someone is following them, acknowledge the paranoia—"It must be difficult to have someone follow you"—but do not tell them they are right or wrong to believe that way.
- If you are accused of something you didn't do, dismiss it calmly and immediately change the subject. If you try to defend yourself, they will take it as proof of your guilt. If they claim something has been stolen, help them look for the object.
- If someone other than yourself is the target, encourage the person to talk about his or her mistrust.
- If you have visitors, explain to them that the person may make false accusations.
- Be aware that crowds can make paranoia worse, and should be avoided by the person who is experiencing these feelings.

HOARDING AND HIDING

Some individuals with Alzheimer's hoard or hide their own possessions in an apparent attempt to hold on to something familiar. Others gather items that belong to their caregiver or other family members. "I called my sister and asked her to help me find my keys," said Virginia. "My husband hid them, and I couldn't find them for five days. He doesn't even remember that he hid them. I thought I had looked everywhere. My sister found them in a flowerpot. I was distraught, but what could I do? Now I have three sets of keys for the house and the car, and I keep them separate. My sister keeps a spare set for me too."

What may appear to be intentional and malicious behavior may in fact be a way for people with Alzheimer's to act out fears and memory loss. Virginia's husband simply forgot where he put down the keys, and questioning him did no good because he didn't remember picking up the keys in the first place.

If the person you are caring for is hiding and hoarding things, take the following precautions:

• Lock away or remove money and valuables such as jewelry from your home. Hoarders often do not realize the value of the items they collect and may throw them away or flush them down the toilet.

• Check your wastebaskets before disposing of their contents. Virginia found six silver spoons in the bottom of the trash in the kitchen.

• Common hiding places are under cushions, in bureau drawers or shoes, and under beds. If the individual had a favorite place to hide birthday and Christmas presents in the past, look there as well.

• Once you find a hiding place, check it periodically. Hoarders often keep using the same spot.

• Have a spare set of items such as keys, eyeglasses, and hearing-aid batteries.

• Lock up some areas of the house so that the person will have fewer places to hide things and you will have a secure area.

• Remind yourself that the person with Alzheimer's is not a thief. Hiding and hoarding can be harmless if you take the proper precautions.

SEXUALITY

Sex and intimacy are basic human needs, and the mental and emotional deterioration associated with Alzheimer's disease has varying effects on these needs. Spouses who are caregivers usually find that their sex life deteriorates as the disease runs its course. "Alzheimer's disease has robbed my husband and me of our sex life," said Gerry. "Lester was always a tender, loving husband. I know it's not his fault, but there's no intimacy, no love in our lovemaking. I feel used. And I know that eventually he won't even want the little we share now."

Spouses may feel turned off by their mate now that they have taken on a "parenting" role. Others, like Gerry, are upset by the lack of intimacy and the realization that it will eventually disappear completely. Spouses know that if not now, then in the relatively near future they will no longer share the affection and sexual satisfaction they may have had with their mate prior to the disease. It is important to maintain as much physical contact as possible to convey caring, loving feelings. This may be in the form of hugging, holding hands, massaging, stroking, and patting. Caregivers can seek the advice of a psychotherapist or counselor who is familiar with Alzheimer's disease on how to cope with their feelings of sexual loss.

Although some people with Alzheimer's lose interest in sex early in the course of the disease, others may express more interest or make advances toward people they believe are someone else from their past. "Jack made a pass at one of our neighbors during a neighborhood picnic," said Ruth. "Fortunately I heard what happened and apologized to her immediately. I told her Jack has

Alzheimer's, and she said she understood, that her brother has the disease too. Then I noticed how much she looked like Jack's first wife. That may be what triggered it."

Another aspect of Alzheimer's is that those with the disease may engage in inappropriate sexual behavior, such as masturbating or undressing in public. "My brother was always involved in the community and civic organizations, so many people know him," said Mel. "We were taking him to the park and community events, but we stopped because we never knew when he would start fondling himself. It's hard to see a man who was a pillar of the community act this way, but we know he has no idea what he's doing."

Such behaviors usually are not motivated by sexual desire as much as they are by an internal or external cue. A woman may take off her blouse, for example, because the room is too hot; a man may remove his pants because he needs to use the toilet. Men and women who masturbate may be seeking the good feeling it brings or relieving frustrations. Some men will reach out and touch a woman's breasts or try to hug her because they want attention or comfort.

Regardless of why individuals act out, do not get angry or laugh, even though you may be embarrassed. Quietly tell them that the behavior is not appropriate and lead them to the bathroom or out of the public eye. If the person seems to need affection, try to increase the amount of attention you give him. Hold his hand, give him a hug, or reach out and pat his arm occasionally.

Finally, if men or women with Alzheimer's make inappropriate advances toward their own children, be aware that this is not incestuous behavior. "My daughter and I were both terribly upset when her father tried to fondle her," said Marie. "She ran out of the house. When I called our therapist the next day, he said, 'Realize that your daughter, Carol, probably looks very much like you did when you were her age. That's who your husband probably sees—you, twenty-five years younger.' Now we know we should just gently distract him while Carol leaves the room."

There is no question that Alzheimer's disease takes a terrible toll on the individual's personality, moods, and behaviors. At the same time these changes can be very painful for the caregiver, who continues to live and care for someone who slowly becomes a stranger. It takes a great deal of courage and fortitude to continue in the caregiving role when someone you love and respect becomes a shadow of his or her former self. Your patience, sensitivity, and perhaps most of all a sense of humor can help you through this trying period.

In the next chapter we'll present strategies for handling the physical and personal-hygiene problems that may arise during the course of the disease.

FIVE

Helping with Physical and Personal-Hygiene Problems

" 'Don't tell me what to wear! I like this blouse. Besides, I just had it cleaned, so it's good as new,' That's what my mother told me. But I knew she hadn't taken off her blouse, or pants, for more than two months. The clothes smelled terrible. I couldn't take it anymore. So I decided to do what one of the women in my support group had done: cut her clothes off while she slept. I figured after that I'd deal with getting her into the shower. If anyone had ever told me I'd be doing such a thing, I never would have believed them. Yet there I was, with the scissors, ripping off those smelly clothes."

—Yvonne

As with memory, mood, and behavior problems, the physical symptoms of Alzheimer's disease tend to worsen over time. As damage to the brain increases, people lose part or all of their memory of how to attend to their everyday needs, such as bathing, dressing, and brushing their teeth. They need you to demonstrate these tasks again and again; some you will have to do for them.

Be aware that you and the person you are caring for may feel uncomfortable or embarrassed about your helping with bathroom and other personal activities. Many caregivers experience such feelings initially, and it helps to share your qualms with others in a caregivers' support group (see chapter 12 for resources). Over time many of these same caregivers come to realize that helping with these tasks is an expression of love and concern. "When I thought of my mother as a good person who had brought me much love throughout my life instead of as an old woman who now needed to wear diapers and be fed, I stopped feeling sorry for myself," said Roxanne. "She deserves to have her dignity preserved. I would want as much for myself if I were in her place."

In this chapter you'll learn about the physical problems that develop in Alzheimer's disease, including loss of coordination, incontinence, and need for help with bathing, dressing and undressing, and grooming. You'll also learn how to make the home environment as safe as possible, given the person's current or anticipated physical limitations.

Be aware that helping with the physical problems associated with Alzheimer's disease requires physical as well as emotional strength on your part. You will need to take good care of yourself and ensure that you get adequate rest, eat a balanced diet, and take time for yourself when needed.

CREATING A SAFE ENVIRONMENT

It is never too early to start figuring out ways to change your home environment so that it is safer for the person with Alzheimer's. As the illness progresses, the person is likely to experience loss of coordination—which can result in falls and injuries—and possibly the need for a

HELPING WITH PHYSICAL AND PERSONAL-HYGIENE PROBLEMS | 71

wheelchair. Go through your house and look for potential hazards—clutter, sharp edges on furniture, fragile items that may break if the person falls or leans against them. Other accidents may result if the person forgets how to use appliances, tries to ingest nonfood items such as cleansers or medicine, or has access to weapons, alcohol, or drugs.

However, before you rush out to buy new furniture or redo the walls and floors, assess the individual's needs, your needs, and the current state of the home. Your goals are to make only the modifications that are necessary, keep them simple, and to balance your needs against those of the person with Alzheimer's.

Start with some of the general guidelines that follow. Then, depending on the status of the person you're caring for, consider making the adaptations suggested in the room-by-room safety guide on pages 73–76.

General Safety Guidelines

• Keep your home as neat as possible; clutter and knickknacks are easily knocked over, and may be distracting or disorienting to the person.

• Avoid floral or still-life patterns in wall and floor coverings, upholstery, and draperies. "The wallpaper in my dad's room had a floral design. One morning I noticed a section of the wall was in shreds. He had tried to pick the flowers off the wall using his nails. He didn't realize the flowers weren't real."

• Use natural lighting where possible, and position light sources so as to avoid casting shadows. Dark corners can look like caves or holes to people with Alzheimer's disease.

- Remove throw rugs. Tack down the edges of carpets.
- Secure all electrical and telephone cords.
- Move or rearrange any furniture that hinders walking or a wheelchair.
- Avoid using folding tables and chairs, which the person can trip over or knock over.
- Have a light source near each doorway, or use nightlights.
- Keep medications out of reach or locked away.
- If the person can no longer safely use items such as a sewing machine, power tools, knives, shears, an iron, or a hair dryer, keep them in a locked closet.
- Remove guns or lock them in a closet.
- Remove poisonous plants, such as philodendron and poinsettia.
- Control access to alcohol.
- Lower the temperature on the hot-water heater so that the person cannot accidentally scald himself or herself when turning on the water. People with Alzheimer's may become less sensitive to heat and cold and may not react quickly enough to prevent injury.
- Place a sturdy chair in front of hot radiators to block access to them. Consider placing a gate around a floor furnace.
- Place locks on your main fuse box and controls for the thermostat and hot-water heater.
- Install security locks on windows and balcony doors.
- Hang bells or chimes on doors leading to the outside

so that you will be alerted when the individual goes out the door.

- Remove locks from inside rooms so that the person cannot lock himself or herself in and deny access to you.
- Check fire extinguishers and smoke alarms monthly.
- Keep a list of emergency phone numbers next to each telephone.

A Room-by-Room Safety Guide

Kitchen

- Don't wax linoleum kitchen floors.
- Use pots and pans with handles that don't conduct heat to prevent burns if the person reaches for a hot pot or pan.
- Use splatter screens on the stove.
- Install childproof latches on cabinets and drawers, and tamper-proof stove knobs and water faucets. "Sophie gets up in the middle of the night and looks for a snack. One night she put a pot of soup on the stove and went back to bed," said Hank. "The pot started burning and the smoke alarms went off. I put the fire out with the extinguisher and immediately removed the knobs from the stove, and the next day I bought tamper-proof knobs."
- Use a hot plate, microwave, or toaster oven for cooking when possible. These are safer than conventional range ovens.
- Keep kitchen matches, toothpicks, plastic bags,

bottles of spices, and other small items in the kitchen out of reach.

- Don't put magnets that look like food on the refrigerator. "My husband thought the cookie magnets on the refrigerator door were real," said Connie. "He broke his tooth trying to eat one."

Bathroom

- Install handrails and grab bars in and around the tub. These are available from medical supply houses. Ask your local Alzheimer's Association office for recommendations.
- Use a tub seat or bench in the shower or tub if the person has problems with balance or muscle weakness. The seat should be the same height as a wheelchair, approximately 19 inches. Some tub seats have adjustable legs or back supports. If you cannot get a tub seat, place a sturdy nonrust chair with rubber tips on the legs in the tub or shower stall.
- Place a rubber mat or decals on the tub floor to prevent slipping.
- Replace glass shower doors with a shower curtain.
- Insulate exposed hot-water pipes under the sink to protect the person's legs while sitting.
- Mirrors or glossy surfaces can be frightening to people with Alzheimer's. "My husband hits his reflection in the bathroom mirror," said Grace. "Now I keep the mirror covered."
- Most toilet seats are too low for people who use wheelchairs. Toilet guard rails or an elevated toilet seat can be installed to compensate.

- The ideal height for sinks for individuals who use wheelchairs is twenty-four inches from the floor. Place a regular chair under the sink if there isn't enough room for a wheelchair.

Bedroom

- If your regular bedroom is on the second floor of the house, consider arranging one on the first floor so that the person you're caring for doesn't have to go up and down stairs.
- Falling out of bed is a common problem. Reduce the risk by placing the bed in a corner. Unless the person is completely bedbound, a hospital bed with railings is not recommended because the individual may try to climb out and fall. An alternative is to place a mattress or futon next to the bed, which will reduce the impact if the person falls.
- Make sure the bed is stable, preferably up against a wall. If you are using a hospital bed, lock the brakes.
- Clothing should be hung on rods that are thirty-six inches from the floor so that they are accessible to a person who uses a wheelchair. Shoes and accessories can be placed in shoe bags that hang from the door.
- Place a telephone or emergency buzzer within easy reach of the bed.

Porch or Patio

- Remove storm doors or cover them with protective grillwork so that the person with Alzheimer's does not inadvertently walk into them or put a hand or foot through them.

- Paint steps to a porch or deck in bright contrasting colors so that they are clearly visible. Install a bannister if it appears the person might fall off the side.
- Check for uneven ground, cracked pavement, and any branches the person might trip over.
- Make sure yard furniture is stable.
- Monitor individuals when they go outdoors. They may eat flowers, weeds, or dirt, or trip on uneven ground or stones.

In the Car

- Seat belts are a must when transporting persons with Alzheimer's. Because individuals may try to grab your arm while you drive, have them sit in the backseat.
- Lock the car doors. Some cars have a childproof locking system that prevents the person in the backseat from unlocking doors manually. If not, place heavy tape over knobs and handles the person may tamper with. "We stopped at a red light, and my mother opened the car door and tried to get out. Luckily she had a seat belt on. She got caught in it long enough for me to put the car in park, get to her side, and put her back into the car."
- Some individuals are afraid to get into vehicles, especially the vans that are often used to transport individuals with disabilities to day-care centers. For people in wheelchairs it may help to back them into the van. They may be less frightened if they cannot see they are being put into a confined area.

In addition to safeguarding the environment, it is important to have an emergency plan ready in case something does happen. For example, whom will you call if the person falls and hurts himself? What will you do in case of a fire? If the person misinterprets your attempts to remove him or her from the home and resists you? Prepare for all contingencies and discuss your plans with other family members and friends.

LOSS OF COORDINATION

The person with Alzheimer's can experience loss of coordination in the hands, fingers, arms, and legs for many different reasons, such as lack of exercise, the use of drugs such as tranquilizers or neuroleptics (medicine for seizures), or medical conditions such as Parkinson's disease or arthritis. If you notice that the person is becoming uncoordinated, arrange for him or her to have a complete physical examination to help determine the cause.

"It happened gradually," said Lenny. "Sometimes my dad seemed a little wobbly when he walked. Then he started to be unsteady when he took a bath, and I had to help him in and out of the tub. Soon he was walking with a distinct shuffling motion."

Onset of loss of coordination is gradual for some people, rapid for others. Therefore you cannot assume that because a person can maneuver the stairs today, he or she will be able to do so next week. Eventually loss of coordination affects most or all of the person's daily living skills. "As Debra lost the coordination in her hands, I tried to find ways to make things easier," said her husband, Rick. "I bought pants with elastic waistbands and sneakers with Velcro tabs for her. She has trouble holding a toothbrush, so I wrapped the handle with cloth and tape to make it thicker. The doctor said it was important for her to do things independently for as long as possible."

As a general rule, if the person is struggling, try to give instructions in a calm voice. Tasks are more difficult to perform when there is tension on either person's part. When possible, break down each task into steps, whether it be dressing, grooming oneself, or doing other daily activities. Specific strategies for these areas will be discussed in the following sections of this chapter.

Be aware that adaptive devices such as buttoners or special utensils generally are not recommended for people with Alzheimer's disease. Although such devices may be effective during rehabilitation for people who have had a stroke or other type of brain injury, people with Alzheimer's disease usually cannot learn how to use them.

People with Alzheimer's may also have difficulty maneuvering a walking aid, such as a cane or walker. Talk with your physician or physical therapist about their use.

Furniture, banisters, and hand railings that once were sturdy may weaken under constant pressure or heavy use. Check them periodically. Also remove from traffic areas any antique furniture or pieces that may tip over. "When my husband first had trouble walking, he leaned on the furniture as he made his way across the room. One day he leaned on a table he had used before and it tipped over," said Lucille. "He fell, and although he didn't seem to be hurt, he couldn't get up. He weighs more than two hundred pounds, and I couldn't help him. I had to call our son."

When a person falls, remember the following advice:

- Remain calm. This may be hard to do, but people who have fallen will become more upset if you are upset as well. Talk quietly until both of you are calm.
- Check for visible signs of pain, cuts, and bruises.
- If the person appears to be unhurt and is calm, wait to see if he or she can get up unaided.
- Don't lift the person yourself, or you may cause injuries.
- Call your physician if you think the person has hit his or her head or if you notice signs of swelling, pain, bruises, agitation, or confusion.

Using a Wheelchair

When loss of coordination becomes severe, the person you're caring for may need to use a wheelchair. Wheelchairs may be rented or purchased outright, and they come with an array of features that may help the person with Alzheimer's. Talk with a physical or occupational therapist before making any decisions. Also be sure to check with your insurance company to see whether the cost of a wheelchair is covered. Requirements vary from company to company.

Some special features you might want to consider include the following:

- Brake extension: This detachable rod increases the

leverage of the brake handle so that less strength is required to engage the brake.

- Elevating foot and leg rests: These are helpful for individuals who have swelling in the leg or foot.
- Removable foot and leg rests: During difficult transfers (see below) removable rests allow you to move the wheelchair in closer to the surface to which you are transferring the person.
- Removable arm rests: Sliding transfers are easier if the arm rests can be removed.
- Wheelchair narrower: When this device is turned, the sides of the wheelchair compress to allow the chair to go through an otherwise impassable doorway. This may cause some pressure on the person's hips, but it is only momentary. After the chair clears the doorway, the chair returns to its original width.

Before you rent or purchase a wheelchair, measure all the doorways in your home. Bathroom doorways are usually the narrowest, thus the chair should fit through this opening. Sometimes the bathroom door and the surrounding molding may need to be removed to permit wheelchair access. A curtain or accordion door can be installed in their place.

Here are additional suggestions to help you plan for wheelchair use:

- You may need a ramp in order to wheel the chair in and out of your home. Commercial ramps are available from home health stores, but these can be expensive. Homemade ramps can be made of plywood and covered with a nonskid material such as indoor/outdoor carpeting. The ramp should be built on a ratio of 12 inches of length per 1 inch of height. That means that if the top step into the front of the house is 30 inches high, the ramp should be 360 inches (30 feet) long. The recommended width is 4 feet.

- Check potential wheelchair routes through your home, and note corners or sharp turns. You may need to move some furniture to permit safe maneuvering through the house.
- Make sure there are no breakable or valuable items along the wheelchair route. Sometimes people may inadvertently push the wheelchair into furniture or grab for items left within reach as they go by.
- Be aware that you may need to secure the individual into the wheelchair when you take him or her outside. "I hated the idea of strapping my wife into her wheelchair," said Stewart. "Then one day we went to the mall, and I turned my back for a minute. She tried to get up and fell. Fortunately she wasn't hurt, but it convinced me to make sure she's secure before I take her out again."

Helping with Transfers

Transfers involve moving the person from one seat or area to another, that is from wheelchair to commode or from wheelchair to car seat. They are necessary when the person loses coordination and muscle strength, generally in the later stages of disease. The two types of transfers you are likely to be involved with are the sliding-board transfers and the lift transfer.

In the sliding-board transfer you slide the person across a smooth two-foot-long board, which bridges the two seats or areas (e.g., from wheelchair to car seat or from wheelchair to toilet seat).

In the lift transfer you lift the person from one place to another, taking care to protect yourself from injury in the process. A physical therapist, occupational therapist, or nurse can show you how to do transfers safely. You should also observe the following guidelines. Even if the person appears capable of doing the transfer by himself or herself, you will need to be ready in the event the transfer isn't successful. This means you may suddenly have the individual's full body weight thrown against you, or you may have to catch the person before a fall.

- Always stand with your knees bent, with a feeling that your weight is centered in your lower body. If you are lifting or moving the individual yourself, the majority of your work should be done by your quadriceps, the big muscles in the tops of your thighs, not your arms and upper or lower back.
- Prepare for the transfer. Talk to the person while moving him or her, saying what you are going to do before you do it and asking for his or her cooperation.
- If the transfer involves a wheelchair, make sure the brake is on, arm and foot rests are out of the way, and clothing is not caught on the chair.
- When possible, the surface you are transferring to and the one you are transferring from should be approximately the same height. It takes extra strength and practice to move someone from a lower to a higher level.
- Make sure the two surfaces are as close together as possible.

INCONTINENCE

Incontinence—the loss of control of one's bladder, bowels, or both—is common in people with Alzheimer's. It has several causes: People can forget when they last went to the bathroom. They may not associate the full feeling in their bladder or colon as a signal to use the toilet. Others cannot find the bathroom, or they forget how to use a toilet. During the early stages of the disease, bladder and bowel incontinence may be caused by drugs, an infection, or stress, and may be temporary. In later stages, however, incontinence usually becomes a permanent condition.

"Accidents happen; that's what I keep telling myself. But we have it pretty much under control," Roy said. During the day Roy reminds his wife to go to the bathroom every two hours. If they go out, he brings along a female relative or friend who can take her into the rest room. "At night she occasionally has a problem," he said. "I restrict her liquid intake after dinner, but sometimes she wakes up and has to urinate. I leave lights on, but if she is frightened, she wets herself. Now I put protective pads on her at night."

Taking care of toilet needs is a private matter; thus, as noted earlier, helping people who have forgotten good habits or who can't communicate their needs can be embarrassing for both you and them. You may feel angry and upset when you have to lead the person to the bathroom and encourage him or her to urinate or defecate. Changing soiled undergarments and helping individuals wipe themselves are tasks most people thought they gave up after taking care of their babies. Many caregivers find that sharing their feelings with others like themselves helps them deal with the discomfort or disgust they feel.

"One woman in my support group told me she imagines herself in her husband's shoes," said Loretta. She told me, 'If anyone had to take care of my personal needs, who better than my husband? Who knows me better than he does? Who knows him better than I do?'"

Urinary Incontinence

Bladder incontinence usually appears before bowel incontinence and is easier to control. If wetting happens occasionally, it may actually be "dribbling"—the leakage of urine that commonly occurs in elderly persons when they exercise, stand up or move quickly, or cough. Note when wetting occurs to see if this is the case.

Other factors that cause or contribute to urinary incontinence include the following:

- A preexisting condition, such as Parkinson's disease, diabetes, or stroke
- Emotional stress: Is a particular situation or environment making the person anxious or agitated?
- Medications, such as sedatives, diuretics, and tranquilizers
- Beverages with a diuretic effect, such as coffee, tea, grapefruit juice, and colas
- Inability to reach the toilet, either because the person is confused, disoriented, or physically unable to maneuver to the bathroom in time

Bowel Incontinence

Once bowel incontinence develops, it is usually irreversible. An exception is fecal impaction (partial or total blockage of the bowels), which occasionally occurs in early Alzheimer's and is treatable. Contact your physician immediately if you notice bowel incontinence.

Privacy and comfort are essential for individuals who have incontinence, but especially bowel incontinence. They will require more time to sit on the toilet, alone or with minimal supervision if possible. To be sure they are safe, install hand rails next to the toilet. If they are restless or upset, play music or read to them (from outside an ajar door) while you monitor them.

What to Do About Incontinence

The following suggestions can help make dealing with incontinence easier for you and the person for whom you are caring:

- Help the person find the bathroom more easily. Tape a picture of a toilet on the bathroom door and tape arrows on the walls to lead the way. Keep a light on at night.
- Have the person wear clothing that is easy to remove, such as pants and skirts with elastic waistbands, to prevent fumbling with buttons and zippers.
- Establish a routine for toileting. This can greatly reduce accidents and the need for protective pads. If the person has urinary incontinence, take him or her to the bathroom every two to three hours and limit liquid intake in the evening. For people with bowel incontinence,

try to follow the elimination routine used in the past, and take them to the toilet at that time.

- Note behaviors that may indicate the individual needs to go to the bathroom. "My mother gets up suddenly and paces when she needs to use the toilet," said Monica. Other clues may be restlessness, clutching at the groin area, or making sounds or facial expressions of discomfort or pain.

- Absorbent pads or protective pants can be worn at night or during the day when a toileting schedule is not successful. These can be purchased at drug and medical supply stores. Consult with your pharmacist or physician about the best items to buy and their proper use.

- For individuals who are bedbound, a waterproof mattress pad along with incontinence pads are necessary. Always keep a layer of cloth between the person's skin and any rubber or plastic sheets and pads. If these synthetic materials come into contact with the skin, they can promote moisture and lead to irritation.

- Good hygiene is vital; deposits of urine and fecal matter can cause infections, pressure sores, and odors. Dispose of soiled pads promptly. After washing the affected skin thoroughly, apply a soothing powder or ointment and fasten a fresh pad.

- Praise individuals when they use the toilet successfully, and never yell at them when they do not. "I reward Olive with peppermint candies when she goes in the toilet," said her sister, Victoria. "If she has an accident, I tell her it's okay, but I don't give her any candy."

CONSTIPATION

Constipation can have various causes and in turn can trigger other problems, such as nausea, headache, stomach pain, and loss of appetite. Lack of exercise, poor nutrition (i.e., too little fiber in the diet, inadequate fluid intake), and medications (i.e., ibuprofen, allopurinol, codeine, amitriptyline, and over-the-counter antacids that contain aluminum or calcium) can cause constipation.

The following suggestions can help take care of constipation:

• Increase the amount of natural fiber in the person's diet to include foods such as apples, beets, corn, grits, lentils, oatmeal, prunes, whole-grain breads, mangoes, potatoes in their skins, and strawberries. This is easier in the earlier stages of the disease, when chewing and swallowing are generally not problems. Nutrition is discussed in more detail in chapter 7.

• Foods that ferment quickly in the stomach, such as sauerkraut, sourdough bread, and cabbage juice, are natural laxatives. For individuals who can tolerate these foods, a mixture of half tomato juice and half sauerkraut juice can be effective. Other natural laxatives include yogurt, cabbage and leafy green vegetables, rhubarb, apricots, and bran products.

• Foods that cause constipation should be avoided: chocolate, cottage cheese, rice, bananas, and refined grain products, such as white bread.

• Encourage the person to drink water, preferably eight glasses a day.

• Daily exercise naturally stimulates the bowels.

- Massaging the abdomen in slow, deep, circular motions helps some individuals.

BATHING

"Bath time is battle time" say many caregivers. If the person seems afraid or resistant to bathing, the first thing to do is to try to determine the reason. Is the person depressed? Does he or she have a physical illness or infection? Is the person sensitive about having someone else in the bathroom? Is the room temperature or water temperature too hot or too cold? Is the person afraid of running water or soap (this often happens with people with Alzheimer's, though the reason why is unclear). Determining the answers to these questions can put you in a better position to manage the bathing routine.

Baths rather than showers are recommended for people with Alzheimer's. Caregivers can assist people who are sitting in a tub or on a shower chair more easily than those standing in a shower, where they also are more likely to slip and fall. Showers can also be frightening, even for those who have always preferred them.

To make bathing as pleasant and safe as possible, several things should be considered. The most important is safety: The bath stall needs to be equipped with grab bars, safety mats, and handrails. Ask a therapist or nurse to show you how to use these devices and how properly to assist a person in and out of the tub.

Preparing and Giving a Bath

Individuals who resist taking a bath need to be approached in a calm but firm manner. For example Stella goes through the same routine every two days when her husband takes his bath. After the water is drawn, she hands him a robe and towel and says "Your bath is ready, Martin." He always counters with "I'm not getting wet, no way." She then proceeds to ask him for his shirt, shoes, socks, pants, and underwear. After every request he says "Not getting wet, no way." She continually refocuses his attention on the next task rather than acknowledge his protests. "If I were to counter his protests with 'Yes you are going to get wet' or 'Yes you will take a bath,' we'd have a battle on our hands," said Stella. "I talk all the way through the bath—'Step into the tub, wash this leg, wash this arm'—until he's done!"

Follow these guidelines when giving a bath:

- Always test the temperature of the water before the individual gets into the tub. People with Alzheimer's often cannot judge temperature.
- Fill the tub with only about three inches of water to avoid possible drowning.
- Assist the person onto a safety bench or into the tub.
- Give him soap-on-a-rope or a washcloth with a soap pocket in it so that he won't drop the bar.
- Never leave the individual unattended. Here you must balance the right of privacy with the need for safety. People who can bathe themselves with little or no help should be allowed to do so. Place a chair outside the bathroom door and supervise from a distance.
- Have towels and a bathrobe ready for after the bath.

Be sure the person is completely dry. Offer a moisturizer or powder.

- Bath time is a good opportunity to check individuals for sores or infections.
- Establish a routine time for bathing and stay with it. "I bathe my brother every morning before I leave for work," said Joan. My sister stays with him during the day. One week I had to go into the office early every day, so I tried to give him a bath at night. He became agitated and wouldn't get into the tub. The next morning he wouldn't eat and he threw his food. I decided it was worth getting up earlier the rest of the week to give him his bath rather than disrupt his routine."

Once individuals reach the stage where they can no longer bathe themselves, you may need to have someone help you—a family member or home health aide—especially if the individual is too large or heavy for you to assist alone. If you can get help only periodically, you might consider giving the person a sponge bath every day and a regular tub bath when you have help.

Dealing with Embarrassment

As noted earlier, bathing and elimination are very personal activities, and caregivers are often uncomfortable with this task. An especially sensitive area is ensuring genital cleanliness. Although distasteful or uncomfortable for many people, cleaning the genital area is very important because this area can harbor infection and produce unpleasant odors. The area under women's breasts is another sensitive spot.

"My father won't wash himself anymore. When I try

to do it for him, he pushes my hands away, especially when I try to do his genitals," said Tom. "A woman in my support group suggested I distract him by getting him to sing. She said, 'Start singing and get him to join in. It might divert his attention long enough to get through at least part of the bath.' It works fairly well. I'm less apprehensive about bathing him now."

Another option is to give the person toys to play with during a bath. Not everyone agrees this is appropriate for adults, but some caregivers find it works very well. Says Charles, whose wife plays with plastic boats while she's in the tub, "Vivian no longer fights me when it's time for her bath. She enjoys herself. I don't think it's infantile at all. Heck, we're never too old to have a little fun, are we?"

Using bubble bath can add a pleasant, sweet-smelling touch. Be cautious, however; some bubble bath is irritating or can make the tub slippery.

People who are reluctant or refuse to get completely undressed may feel more comfortable wearing a towel draped over their shoulders or wearing their underwear in the tub.

DRESSING AND UNDRESSING

Remember how grown up you felt when you learned how to dress yourself? Now imagine how it feels to have forgotten how to button a shirt or put on a pair of pants. "My brother put his pants on, then his underwear on top," said Walter. "I have to stay with him and hand him each piece of clothing. I can't just leave everything on the bed and let him do it himself."

Helping people with Alzheimer's disease get dressed and dressing them yourself are two different approaches to the same goal: making sure they are clothed in comfort and with dignity. Allow the person to do as much on his or her own as possible. This helps maintain the person's sense of self-esteem and independence. How much help you actually need to offer will depend on the degree of impairment of the person's memory, balance, and motor skills.

Be aware that people with Alzheimer's often do not recognize their own clothing or have any sense of which colors look good together. They may want to wear an overcoat in the summer or shorts in the winter. You may need to make choices for them. But until they reach the latter stages of the disease, most individuals with Alzheimer's can dress themselves with your help. The key is to make dressing and undressing as easy and as tension-free as possible for both of you. Follow these guidelines to help with dressing and undressing:

- Separate clothing by type: all sweaters in one drawer, all underwear in another, and so on. Once you've established these locations, don't change them, or you will confuse the person you're caring for.
- Label the drawers with pictures of what they contain.
- Washable, permanent-press clothing presents the least amount of work for you.
- Stay with basic colors and solids. This lessens problems with color coordination.
- Offer the individual limited choices. "I let my mother choose between two dresses or two outfits every day," said Felicia. "She points to the one she wants. She

always took pride in how she dressed. I want her to continue to have a say in how she looks."

- Some individuals, such as Thelma, insist on wearing the same clothes every day. If possible, buy duplicates of these items so that you can launder one set while they wear another.

- Buy clothing that is easy to put on and take off. Buttoning a shirt can be a frustrating task. Pullover sweaters and shirts, pants and skirts with elastic waists, jogging suits, and shoes with Velcro strips are good choices. Clothes with buttons or snaps can be adapted using pressure tape or Velcro.

- Slip-on shoes and sneakers with Velcro closures are the easiest to put on and remove. Crepe soles help to prevent slips and falls.

- Place clothing on the bed in the order it should be put on. Then give simple instructions for each item. "I lay everything out on the bed and then hand my husband each piece," explains Harriet. "Then I tell him when to sit, which leg to put in first, when to stand. Sometimes I demonstrate for him; for example, I'll put on my coat and then he'll put on his.

- As the person undresses, remove from sight anything that needs to be washed. When he or she takes off night clothes, for example, put them away immediately so that he or she won't be tempted to put them back on.

- Routinely inspect the person's clothing for holes, spots, and stains. Some people habitually pick at or rip their clothes.

- Thoroughly check the person's clothing before he or she leaves the house. Is everything clean? Does everything match? Is it appropriate for the weather? Is anything on inside out? "I usually check how my mother is dressed before we go out," Richard said. "One day she came out of her room with her coat already on. I looked down and saw that her shoes were on the proper feet and her slacks were the ones I had put out for her. When we got to my sister's house, Mom took off her coat and she didn't have a blouse on! Lucky it was my sister's house and not the eye doctor's office, which was where we were going!"

GROOMING

Having attractive hair, nails, and skin are an essential part of a person's self-esteem. Although individuals with Alzheimer's eventually seem to lose interest in their appearance, this may result at least in part from their forgetting how to care for themselves. It's important for you, too, that they look their best. It is more pleasant to care for someone who is well groomed than a person who is unkempt and smells bad.

"My mother always wore makeup and had her hair done every week," said Ronni. "Once she stopped taking care of her own appearance, I felt she deserved to keep looking as attractive as she always had. Now we never go out without her wearing makeup and a nice dress. She won't let a hairdresser touch her head, but I brush her hair and put pretty combs in it. Someone once said to me, 'She doesn't look like she has Alzheimer's.' Well, how is she supposed to look? Sloppy and dirty?"

Grooming can be part of a person's daily routine, perhaps done in conjunction with bathing. At a minimum hair should be brushed or combed at least once a day and washed twice a week; hands should be washed before and after meals; skin lotion should be applied to dry areas at least once a day; deodorant should be applied after bathing; and nails should be trimmed as needed. Men often need to shave, and women may shave their legs. If a woman wore makeup in the past, help her apply it now.

As with bathing, allow the person you're caring for to do as much of his or her own grooming as possible, even if the result is a little uneven. You can always tidy up hair or fix makeup after. And remember, a little compliment can go a long way. Tell the person how nice he or she looks, and suggest that other family members and friends comment as well.

Hair

A short, easy-to-manage hairstyle is recommended for men and women. If a trip to the beauty parlor or barbershop is impossible, you may find a beautician or barber who makes house calls. Some caregivers trim the person's hair themselves. Electric clippers are easy to use, but the sound may be disturbing. Safety scissors with rounded tips are best for those who may not sit still for a haircut.

Washing the person's hair when he or she bathes has advantages and disadvantages. If bath time is already an ordeal, adding an extra task may be too tiring for you. Physically it may be hard on your back and knees to reach into the tub. A handheld sprayer hose can make this part easier. You may opt to wash the individual's hair in the sink, in which case a sprayer hose can be attached to the sink faucet. A dry shampoo is the easiest and least traumatic approach for individuals who are bedbound. It works nearly as well as soap and water.

Shaving

Shaving is another grooming habit that is important to continue for men with Alzheimer's. "My husband always seems to perk up after I give him a shave," said Harriet. "Even though he can't tell me how he feels, I can sense a difference. Maybe it's the aftershave I put on him. It was always his favorite." Electric razors should be used (the same holds true for women who may wish to shave their legs or underarms).

Skin Care

A massage is an excellent way to improve circulation and skin tone, especially for individuals who are bedridden or wheelchair bound. "My dad can't speak anymore, but when I give him a massage, I can tell by the look in his eyes that he appreciates it," said his daughter, Libby.

Dry skin is always a concern, and daily application of moisturizers and emollients is recommended. Proper nutrition and exercise also promote healthy skin.

Certain areas of the body are prone to harbor moisture and bacteria—the groin, under the breasts in women, and between any folds of skin. Keep these areas dry and clean.

Watch for signs of pressure sores—areas of skin where constant pressure has caused the surface cells to die and wear away. These sores start as areas of skin that look tender, pink or red, and slightly warm to the touch. When you apply pressure, the redness disappears and returns as soon as you release it.

Persons who use wheelchairs are prone to pressure sores on their ankles and heels, back of the knees and thighs, the elbows, and the lower and middle back. For bedridden individuals check their heels, calves, elbows, buttocks, shoulder blades, and back of the head.

To help prevent pressure sores from developing, follow these measures:

- Individuals confined to bed should shift position at least every two hours. Encourage them to roll onto their side or to sit up. A therapist or nurse can show you how to handle people who have physical problems, such as paralysis or a broken hip.
- People who are incontinent (loss of the ability to control urination or bowel movements) need to be kept clean and dry.
- If you find a potential pressure sore, apply a skin ointment and gently rub the area to promote circulation. If the area worsens, call a physician.
- Avoid clothing that is restrictive or that can rub or irritate the skin.

If pressure sores do occur, contact your physician immediately.

Foot and Nail Care

Foot care is easy to overlook because feet are usually out of sight—in shoes or slippers or beneath the bedcovers—and thus out of mind. To ensure proper foot care, keep these tips in mind:

- Inspect the feet when the individual bathes or when you are checking for pressure sores.
- Feet that perspire a lot need to be kept dry. Cotton

socks absorb moisture, and baby or foot powder dusted between the toes can help. If possible, allow the individual to go without shoes for at least an hour a day.

- Avoid use of pantyhose, tight shoes, and tight socks.
- Trim toenails and fingernails every two to three weeks. Be alert for ingrown nails, which can be extremely painful and become infected easily. Keep fingernails short and clean underneath, as some people with Alzheimer's tend to put their fingers into their mouth, which can spread bacteria.

Dental Care

Good oral hygiene is linked directly to nutrition (see chapter 6). When people have tooth or mouth pain from a toothache, infection, gum problems, or ill-fitting dentures, they may stop eating, and digestion problems or constipation may develop. To prevent these situations, individuals need to brush their teeth or clean their dentures every day. These can seem like insurmountable tasks for people with Alzheimer's. You may have to show them step-by-step how to open the toothpaste, put it on the bristles, and how to brush.

"Tony would not brush his teeth or let me do it for him. He clenched his mouth shut like a steel trap," said Nora. "So I put toothpaste on his brush and mine, gave him his brush, and started brushing my own teeth. He just watched me until I took his hand and moved it up and down in front of his mouth. Then he got it. Now we brush our teeth together."

Routine dental appointments should be kept if at all possible. At-home dental care should include the following:

- Dentures should be removed and cleaned daily, and the gums should be checked for irritation. Even small sores can lead to big problems, especially since individuals with Alzheimer's usually cannot tell you how they feel or if something hurts.
- Encourage the person to brush after meals. If he or she can use mouthwash without swallowing it, include this as part of the dental plan. You may need to demonstrate how to spit out the mouthwash.
- Be aware of bad breath. It may signal infection, plaque buildup, or gum disease.
- Do a routine examination for sores, red gums, lesions on the tongue, and tooth decay.
- Check dentures periodically for signs of ill fit and irritation. If you suspect a problem, contact a dentist.

Makeup

Women who always wore makeup will likely appreciate help in this area. Men who are embarrassed or apprehensive about helping them with makeup can ask a female relative or friend to do it for them. Allowing women with Alzheimer's to present their best face to the world is a wonderful boost to their morale. "Gladys wore makeup nearly every day of our married life. Lately she gave up trying to put it on," said Victor. "When her sister, Iris, visits us once a week, she makes Gladys up. Gladys notices, because she smiles at herself in the mirror. Now Iris showed me how to put lipstick on Gladys. It's not much, but it makes Gladys smile."

Helping the person with Alzheimer's feel safe and comfortable at home, and appropriately dressed and groomed for social interactions, can be a challenge for even the most committed caregiver. The person you are caring for may resist all efforts on your part to bathe, dress, or help in other aspects of daily care. You can stay motivated by reminding yourself that your efforts will likely result in the person's ability to maintain a sense of dignity and self-esteem for as long as possible, and this will make you feel better too.

SIX

Your Role in Medical Therapy

"What worries me is that Leo can't tell me when something bothers him. Sometimes he looks like his stomach hurts. I touch his stomach and make a sad face and ask him, 'Does it hurt?' but he doesn't answer me. I can only guess if there's a problem—unless it's obvious, such as a cough or a fever."

—Jenny

As the disease progresses, men and women with Alzheimer's become more susceptible to medical ailments. There are numerous reasons for this: A breakdown in their immune system may leave them more vulnerable to infections; poor nutrition may lead to poor resistance to disease; difficulty in maintaining good hygiene may lead to various types of infections. Some people also have preexisting medical conditions, such as high blood pressure or diabetes, that must continue to be treated during the course of the disease.

With respect to Alzheimer's itself, no medications currently exist to prevent or cure the disease (see chapter 2 for information on participating in clinical trials of experimental treatments). However, some physicians may prescribe drugs to treat some of the symptoms of the disease, such as depression, hallucinations, restlessness, or sleeplessness. These drugs may also cause unwanted side effects that may actually make symptoms worse. For example, some medications can cause the person to become agitated or to have coordination problems or constipation.

This situation has several implications for caregivers. First, it is important to make sure one physician is in charge of coordinating the person's care and monitoring his or her medical problems. In addition, if possible, one pharmacist should be selected to supply needed medications, explain how and when they should be administered, and help avoid drug interactions. Finally, you will need to become familiar with the person's medical problems and medications, coordinate pill-taking regimens, and keep an eye out for signs of drug side effects or symptoms that indicate a given disorder may be worsening and require immediate professional attention.

Although so much responsibility may seem daunting, this chapter can help. We'll provide tips on how to select a coordinating physician and pharmacist as well as other health professionals, and how to manage medications. Plus, we'll take a look at some of the symptoms of Alzheimer's disease and their treatment.

SELECTING A PHYSICIAN TO COORDINATE CARE

The disease course can run up to twenty years or more, so it is important that you select a physician you like and trust. This physician need not be the one who gave the diagnosis of Alzheimer's, nor does it have to be a specialist. However, he or she should meet the following requirements:

- Have a knowledge and understanding of Alzheimer's disease and delirium and of the medications to treat secondary symptoms.
- Have the time and inclination to listen to you and the person with Alzheimer's and address your questions and concerns. "I told one doctor I wanted to have my husband and son join in on the discussions about my mother. He said that wasn't necessary, that he only needed to talk to me. That's when I knew I wasn't going to talk to him. Our whole family is involved in caring for my mother, and I want a doctor who is concerned about all of us."
- Be easily accessible and have a qualified colleague who takes over when he or she is out of reach.
- Refer you to physical therapists, occupational therapists, psychiatrists, and social workers who can address specific needs.

Ideally the one who coordinates the person's medical care would be your family physician—a general practitioner or internist who knows the person's medical history and personality before developing the disease.

However, it's possible that you don't have such a doctor now. Although many families used to have a family physician who followed them over many years, the dramatic changes that have taken place in our health care system in recent years have changed this situation for many people.

Today you may belong to a managed-care system or have a health care plan that permits you to choose from among a small pool of member physicians rather than selecting from among all physicians. If this is the case for you, then your choices may be limited. Nevertheless most health care plans do permit you at least some choice. So, if you don't feel comfortable with your present physician, you should exercise your right to make other choices.

When seeking a new physician, compile a list of doctors whose work is praised by people you respect—friends, family members, community leaders, other health care workers, other physician specialists. You may also consult the *Dictionary of Medical Specialists,* which is available at your local library. Look for a neurologist or general practitioner experienced in caring for the elderly.

Often recommendations from other caregivers offer the most insight. For example, Beatrice recalls that someone in her support group recommended Dr. M. because "although others are probably equally qualified, Dr. M. always had his nurse call me if the doctor's appointments were running late. We never sit in the waiting room for more than ten minutes. Consideration like that means a lot when you're caring for a person with Alzheimer's."

Next set up consultation appointments with each prospective physician. Be prepared to pay a fee, usually equal to the fee of a standard office visit. When setting the consultation appointment, get as much information as you can about how the doctor runs the practice, including office hours, waiting time for appointments, and payment schedule. In addition to getting helpful information, asking questions permits you to assess the cordiality and professionalism of the office staff.

Following are some tips for finding the best possible

physician to coordinate the person's care and be available to respond to your questions and concerns. When you have narrowed your selection to one or two physicians, consider bringing the person with Alzheimer's with you to an interview to see how he or she and the physician interact.

What to Look for in a Physician: A Checklist

A good physician provides you with information in a forthright way, treats you with respect and concern, and has an office staff that is efficient and friendly. It's best to "doctor shop" as early in the disease process as possible, but it's never too late to change if you feel your current physician is not meeting your needs. The following checklist provides you with questions to ask yourself during the selection process:

Does the doctor . . .

_____Communicate with me in a way I can understand without being condescending? Allow me to express fears about the person's symptoms or certain forms of treatment? Give me real information about the person's condition instead of a simple pat on the back and reassurance?

_____Seem knowledgeable about Alzheimer's, including the latest treatment options for specific symptoms?

_____Explain medical tests and procedures before performing them? Discuss potential side effects or complications?

_____Take time to answer my questions and those of the person with Alzheimer's without rushing us?

_____Talk with the individual as a person before beginning an examination? Treat us courteously and with respect?

_____Behave in an authoritarian way? Or in an easygoing manner?

_____Seem comfortable with the idea of my getting a second opinion? Or threatened and defensive?

_____Have a staff that is efficient and friendly?

_____Have regular office hours during the day, evenings, and on weekends? Have a backup physician when he or she is not available?

_____Regularly keep to the appointment schedule instead of keeping us waiting for long periods in the waiting room?

_____Permit me to pay over time when visits aren't covered by insurance?

_____Permit me to pay by check or credit card?

SELECTING OTHER HEALTH PROFESSIONALS

The same criteria described above may be used to select other health professionals, such as a physical therapist, social worker, or psychologist. However, it is particularly important that the person with Alzheimer's feel comfortable with a specialist, especially if he or she will see the person on a regular basis. If possible, bring the person with you to the interviews and permit him or her to become involved in the selection process.

Selecting a Pharmacist

A pharmacist, like any other health professional, should be chosen with care. Registered pharmacists have special training and education in pharmaceuticals—prescription and over-the-counter drugs. As noted earlier, they are often in the best position to talk about potential side effects of medication, possible interactions among various medicines the person may be taking, how often to take a particular medicine, whether to have it before or with meals, and any other issues pertaining to the medicines the person may be taking for Alzheimer's-related problems and other medical conditions. Although these concerns should also be discussed with a physician, a physician may not be aware of all aspects of importance for each and every medication. That is the responsibility of the pharmacist.

Like a good physician, a good pharmacist should be willing to respond to your questions and concerns. The pharmacist can also act as a medication coordinator, staying alert to possible adverse interactions, expired prescriptions, and so on. Many pharmacies today have computerized records for each customer, noting all the medications he or she is taking (assuming, of course, that you purchase them in the same pharmacy). Some also have computer software that automatically alerts them to potential drug interactions when an additional medicine is prescribed.

If the person has chronic conditions that require treatment over long periods of time, it's in both of your best interests to make friends with a pharmacist and take advantage of his or her specialized knowledge. The way to tell whether a pharmacist will be responsive to your needs is to ask questions and gauge his or her willingness to respond candidly and helpfully.

Of course cost of medication is also an important factor. You probably won't want to patronize a pharmacy that consistently offers products at higher prices than other nearby pharmacies. However, once you establish a relationship with a pharmacist where medications are competitively priced, if you happen to see a product advertised for less at a competing pharmacy, you may ask if your pharmacist will meet that price.

A WORD ABOUT LIFESTYLE

In this chapter we will emphasize the importance of medication in treating some of the symptoms of Alzheimer's, as well as some preexisting medical conditions. However, in many cases lifestyle changes should be tried before medication when possible. For example, proper diet and regular exercise, as well as quitting smoking, can help lower blood pressure and reduce gastrointestinal problems and limit the need for medication.

Stress-reduction techniques such as visualization and meditation can be helpful in reducing the tension and anxiety that may lead to inappropriate behaviors or depression. In some cases they may also reduce pain by helping the person to relax.

Of course other conditions such as edema (swelling), blood clots, and seizures will require medication. Medication will also be necessary if lifestyle changes are not effective enough, or if the person cannot implement them; for example if the person has very limited mobility, it won't be possible to attain the level of exercise required to lower blood pressure, or if the person has chewing and swallowing problems, then foods high in fiber can't be incorporated into the diet as easily.

DRUGS: WHAT EVERY CAREGIVER SHOULD KNOW

As a caregiver you have the responsibility of watching for and reporting to the physician any side effects, behavior changes, and symptoms that could be associated with the person's medications. Being alert to side effects is particularly important when the person has difficulty communicating and may not be able to let you know how he or she is feeling. Of course if the person is very forgetful and confused, you alone may be responsible for ensuring that the correct medications are taken, in the proper doses.

To become as informed as possible about each medication, ask your physician or pharmacist the following questions. To ensure that you remember all responses, take notes, ask for written instructions, or tape your conversation.

Questions to ask about medications:

- What is this drug supposed to do for the problem?
- What are the side effects, both common and infrequent?
- What time(s) of day should the drug be taken?
- Should the drug be taken with food, before or after meals, or on an empty stomach?
- Should certain foods be avoided while taking this medicine?
- Is the drug available in another form? If it's a tab-

let, can it be ground up and mixed with food? People who have trouble swallowing may find it easier to take a ground-up pill mixed with applesauce, or a liquid form if available.
- Should certain activities be avoided while taking this medicine?
- How long should the medication be taken?
- How long until some benefit will be apparent?
- Might it interact with other drugs the person is taking?

ORGANIZING MEDICINES

"Maryellen is taking four different medications," says her daughter, Carolyn. "Keeping them all straight—correct dosages, when to give them, and special instructions—is confusing. I need an easy and accurate way to handle it."

Carolyn's problem may be solved by using a basic chart that has the following categories:

Name of medication:
Prescribed to treat:
Prescribing physician:
Start date:
Looks like (e.g., pink tablet, white capsule):
When to take:
How to take:
Purchased at:
May renew:

Consider drawing the chart on a large, washable memo board so that you can make changes easily. Keep an extra copy on paper with you for when you visit the doctor.

For people who are only mildly confused, develop a color-coded system. Next to the name of each medication place a large colored sticker that matches one that you place on each dispensing container.

Pills can also be placed in morning, noon, dinner, and bedtime sections to correspond to the time that the pill should be taken. The containers can be filled by the caregiver to be sure the correct dosage is taken at the correct times.

A Word About New Medications

As of this writing, scientists are trying to determine the cause of Alzheimer's disease so that treatments to prevent the disease or halt its course for good may be developed. In the meantime one drug that appears to provide temporary benefits to some people with Alzheimer's has recently been approved. The drug tacrine seems to produce small improvements in thinking skills (2.2 improvement on a scale of 70) in some people with mild to moderate disease. The benefits last only about six months, however; then decline continues. Tacrine may produce side effects that include nausea, vomiting, diarrhea, abdominal pain, and liver abnormalities. The drug costs about $112 per month, and blood tests to monitor for liver abnormalities may cost another $148 per month, according to one of the researchers. Talk with your physician to see whether tacrine is an option for the person you're caring for.

Other medications that may produce temporary benefits are being explored in animal models. If these drugs are deemed promising, they may ultimately be tried in humans (for information on participating in clinical trials of potentially helpful drugs, see chapter 2).

MANAGING MEDICAL PROBLEMS

As a person's communication skills and ability to recognize pain deteriorate, you will need to monitor for signs of pain, illness, or injury. Problems with poor vision or faulty hearing are difficult to detect; is the person not responding because he doesn't understand you or because he can't hear you? Is she bumping into furniture because her coordination is poor or because her sight is worsening?

Sometimes the only clue you will have that something is wrong is a sudden shift in the person's behavior; for example, refusal to eat, even when presented with a favorite food, may indicate a dental or gastrointestinal problem. Other clues to possible medical problems include the following:

- Temperature higher than 100 degrees F (although lack of fever does not mean an individual is well). Liquid-crystal thermometers, which are placed on the skin, are safer to use than oral ones.
- Pale, flushed, or dry skin.
- Sudden increase in or onset of drowsiness, irritability, confusion, or belligerence.
- Swelling, especially of the hands, feet, or legs.
- Pale or bleeding gums.

- Diarrhea or vomiting.
- Yelling or moaning.
- Respiratory problems, such as coughing, sneezing, or shortness of breath.
- Sudden weight loss.

Burns, cuts, bruises, and even broken bones may occur and remain unreported by individuals with Alzheimer's, either because the pain center in the brain has been damaged or because they cannot communicate the problem to anyone. Refusal to use the toilet when there had not been a problem previously may signal the presence of pain, as may increased restlessness, shouting, moaning, crying, and holding parts of the body. If the person cannot tell you what hurts and you cannot determine the cause of the behavior, consult your physician. Roxanne recalls how she found out her mother's toe was broken. "I was giving my mother a bath when I noticed her big toe was black and swollen. For the past two days she had refused to take her slippers off. I hadn't insisted, because I thought her feet were cold." Roxanne immediately took her mother to the doctor. "The toe was broken," Roxanne said. "I don't know how she did it, but the doctor said it didn't look like she had dropped anything on it. She may have kicked a wall or just stubbed it real hard. But she can't tell me what happened."

Finally, remember that people with Alzheimer's can be in pain from little things too. Shoes can be too tight, clothes can rub the skin raw, dentures may be fitted poorly, or a ring can cut off circulation. If it can hurt you, it can hurt them.

On the following pages we will review the medical treatment of common problems and symptoms experienced by people with Alzheimer's, including pain, swelling, pressure sores, seizures, and mood problems—and what you can do to help. We'll also look briefly at the treatment for related medical problems, and what to do if hospitalization is required.

Pain

Alzheimer's disease is not a painful illness, but individuals with it do experience some painful conditions, some of which are indirectly related to Alzheimer's. "Miranda scalded her hand in the bathroom sink and she didn't even complain!" said her husband. "She was treated for second-degree burns. Yet last week she bumped her leg on the coffee table, and she cried for twenty minutes. It wasn't much more than a tap, so I think she was frightened more than hurt. It's hard to believe she could feel the bump but not the burn."

Some people are like Miranda who, once they reach the moderate or advanced stages of the disease, cannot discriminate between hot and cold. Others, like Roxanne's mother, may have a reduced sense of pain or simply be unable to tell you that they have been hurt. This is why it is important to pay attention to clues that may indicate pain, such as a sudden worsening of behavior, increased restlessness, or refusal to do certain activities.

Two types of medicines are generally prescribed to treat pain. One type, called *narcotic analgesics,* are powerful painkillers and would be prescribed only when the person is in severe pain that is not relieved by other measures. Side effects of these morphine-derived drugs include nausea, vomiting, gastrointestinal upset, dizziness, drowsiness and fatigue, constipation, and in some cases risk of dependency.

The other category of pain medication is called the *nonsteroidal anti-inflammatory drugs (NSAIDs)*. These include over-the-counter medicines such as ibuprofen. Although some NSAIDs are available over the counter, they should not be self-prescribed. Always consult your physician before giving the person in your care pain medicine—or any type of medicine. Possible side effects of NSAIDs include loss of appetite, bloating, and headache. The possibility of side effects may be reduced if NSAIDs are taken with food or milk.

In addition to drug treatment the severity of pain may be reduced if the individual is relaxed and comfortable. Reducing stimuli, playing soothing music, and generally creating a calm atmosphere can often help.

Edema

Edema is swelling of the feet, legs, or other body parts due to decreased blood circulation, general lack of mobility, kidney or bladder disturbances, or diabetes. It is especially common in people with Alzheimer's who spend much of their time in bed or in a wheelchair.

Diuretics are commonly prescribed for this condition. These agents decrease excess fluid in the body by increasing urine output. Commonly prescribed diuretics include, among others, Midamor, Bumex, and Lasix. These drugs may cause the following side effects:

- Fall in blood pressure
- Rash
- Photosensitivity—when the skin becomes abnor-

mally sensitive to sunlight, and brief exposure can cause rashes
- Nausea and vomiting
- Headache
- Dizziness or fainting
- Leg cramps
- Dehydration and electrolyte imbalances
- Increased blood sugar

Along with drug treatment edema may be treated by elevating the swollen limb above the heart level and increasing the amount of movement in general (see chapter 8 for more information on exercise).

Pressure Sores

Pressure sores are ulcers that develop on the skin of people who are bedridden or immobile for extended periods, such as those in wheelchairs. The sores start as red, painful areas that become purple before the skin breaks down, developing into open sores that may become large, infected, and slow to heal. Pressure sores should be checked out by a physician or nurse. Those that are not infected can be treated with dressings, creams, or powders. If infection sets in, antibiotics may be prescribed.

Sleep Disturbances

Sleeplessness can have various causes. Besides the popular observation that many older people don't seem to need as much sleep as younger people do, individuals with Alzheimer's may have sleep problems because the portion of the brain that regulates sleep is damaged, or they may have dreams that disturb them.

"Roger sleeps for about three hours and then gets up and wanders around the house," said Natalie. "Then I have to make him hot milk because I'm afraid to let him do it himself. Sometimes playing the radio or watching TV puts him back to sleep. But it takes me a long time to fall back to sleep, and I wake up exhausted."

Lack of sufficient physical activity and napping during the day can also prevent individuals from feeling tired enough to sleep at night. Participation in adult-day-care or other activities may offer them the exercise they need. For example Natalie's physician suggested she and Ron take a walk before dinner every night. After doing that for several days Ron started sleeping a few hours longer. Natalie then got an exercise videotape, and now she and Ron do stretching exercises before going to bed at night. "It relaxes both of us," she said. "We're both getting more sleep nowadays."

Finding the cause of sleeplessness is important for you as well as for the person with Alzheimer's. Not only is your sleep disturbed but you probably won't have an opportunity to "catch up" on lost sleep during the day. Continuous lack of sufficient sleep places significant stress on your emotions and health. Talk with your physician about other potential causes of sleeplessness, including the following:

- Sleeplessness may be a side effect of medication the person is taking for a medical condition. For example, diuretics prescribed to treat edema may cause sleep disturbances. Discuss this possibility with your physician or pharmacist.

- Medical conditions such as diabetes, alcoholism, heart disorders, urinary tract infections, and ulcers can all cause sleeplessness. Or the person may be suffering from arthritis pain, or leg cramps, or have breathing difficulties. A complete physical exam may be needed.
- Depression can cause people to routinely wake up very early (two or four o'clock in the morning). If they are taking antidepressants, dosing at bedtime may help them sleep.
- Waking in the middle of the night to use the bathroom can also cause sleep disturbances. This experience can also be frightening for people who are confused. Encourage toilet use before going to bed. Use reflector tape on the floor or wall to mark the way to the bathroom. Leave night-lights on in the bedroom, hallway, and bathroom.
- Caffeine (soft drinks, coffee, tea, chocolate) consumption during the day can trigger sleeplessness at night. Switch to decaffeinated coffee and tea.
- Hunger pangs may cause sleeplessness. Offer the person a light snack before bedtime. Low- or no-fat calcium products (warm low-fat milk, yogurt) or herbal tea may be soothing.
- Make the bed and the bedroom comfortable. Play soft music on a radio next to the bed. Make sure the person is comfortably warm (or cool, in warm weather).
- Once you establish bedtime and waking times, maintain the routine as much as possible.

Drugs that induce sleep, such as diphenhydramine and trazadone, should be used only under a doctor's supervision. Some people with Alzheimer's who take sleeping pills become more confused and anxious. Therefore try all other approaches before you consider drugs.

Depression

Depression is a fairly common response to a diagnosis of Alzheimer's (see chapter 1). "I was devastated to learn my wife had Alzheimer's," said Sam. "But not as devastated as she was. Ethel went into a deep depression and wouldn't talk to anybody. She stayed in bed day in and day out for more than a week. Finally, I convinced her to get up, get dressed, and go to the doctor. He spent about half an hour talking with Ethel and also referred both of us to a counselor. We went to weekly sessions for about six months, and it helped a lot. As it turns out, Ethel's condition hasn't changed much in the past two years, so we still enjoy a pretty active social life, even now."

While depression may be more common in the early stages of disease, it can happen at any time. The causes of depression are not well understood. Certainly deep sadness about having a chronic illness can lead to depression. But chemical changes in the brain may also be a cause.

In general, before prescribing drugs many physicians will suggest a person make lifestyle changes (e.g., more physical activity and social interaction), or try psychotherapy or counseling. If these strategies don't work, antidepressants such as Elavil or Asendin may be prescribed. However, these medications can cause side effects such as drowsiness and fatigue, loss of coordination, dizziness, nausea, blurred vision, and dysphagia (difficulty in swallowing), and for some people the benefits of medication often must be weighed against the drawbacks of side effects.

Aggression and Agitation

If the person you're caring for is aggressive or agitated, the nondrug strategies described in chapter 4 should be attempted. For severe mood and behavior problems that don't respond to behavioral strategies, antianxiety agents, such as Xanax (alprazolam) and Librium (chlordiazepoxide), may be prescribed. Possible side effects of these drugs include sedation, dry mouth, blurred vision, nightmares, increased confusion, headache, constipation, and involuntary twitches and lip smacking. Sometimes switching from one drug to another can reduce unwanted side effects.

Hallucinations

Hallucinations are perceptions of things, sounds, smells, tastes, or physical sensations that are not really there. As noted in chapter 4, some hallucinations may result from treatable conditions such as drug or alcohol abuse, dehydration, bladder or kidney infections, or intense pain. Therefore the first thing to do if the person you're caring for hallucinates is to schedule an appointment with your physician for a complete physical examination. If the nondrug strategies suggested in chapter 4 are not effective, your physician may prescribe an antipsychotic or antianxiety drug to calm the person.

Seizures

Seizures—sudden episodes of uncontrolled electrical activity in the brain that may cause tingling or twitching of an area of the body, hallucinations, fear, or other intense feelings—are not common in people with Alzheimer's disease. When they do occur, they may be associated with other conditions (fever or cerebral injury, for example) and not Alzheimer's.

"No one ever warned me Powell could have a seizure," said Madeline. "I called the emergency medical team right away. The dispatcher kept telling me to stay calm, that Powell would be okay. But I felt as though my heart were in my throat. I guess the seizure only lasted a minute or so; it was over by the time the team arrived. But I never want to go through that again."

The type of seizure most people are familiar with is the generalized tonic-clonic seizure where people become rigid, fall, and lose consciousness. The muscles jerk for about ten to twenty seconds and the teeth may be clenched. Then the person regains consciousness slowly and may have a headache or be confused and sleepy. Other seizures may appear simply as repetitive twitching in an arm or a leg and are called partial seizures. Although seizures are frightening, they are rarely life-threatening.

If the person you are caring for has a tonic-clonic seizure, take the following steps:

- Remain calm. Do not try to restrain the person.

- Make the area safe by moving objects out of the way that may harm the person.
- Stay with the person, but don't try to put a spoon in his or her mouth. Contrary to popular belief, biting the tongue is rare during a seizure; no attempt should be made to prevent it by wedging the mouth open. You can loosen clothing, such as a belt or buttons on a shirt or pants. Let the seizure run its course.
- After the seizure has stopped, allow the person to sleep.
- Call your physician or 911.

If the possibility of recurrent seizures exists, an anticonvulsant such as Dilantin or Tegretol may be prescribed. Side effects from such medications may include nausea and vomiting, diarrhea or constipation, lethargy, depression, or confusion.

Vision Problems

People with Alzheimer's experience the normal deterioration of vision that often accompanies age, including the development of cataracts, but they may also have additional difficulties. "Martin has always worn glasses. I noticed he was fishing around for the food on his plate, and he also seemed to be straining to see when he walked through the apartment."

Stella took her husband to his regular ophthalmologist, but when the trouble was dismissed as "old age," she wasn't satisfied. "I took him to an ophthalmologist who works with Alzheimer's patients. He explained how people with Alzheimer's often have trouble with depth perception and distinguishing between similar colors."

The doctor prescribed bifocals and suggested that Stella paint doorways and railings in her apartment a contrasting color. "All the walls and trim in the apartment are ivory," she said. "I got permission from the management to paint the doorways to Martin's room beige with brown trim. It's helped him quite a bit."

Like Martin many people with Alzheimer's can't distinguish colors well. They may also have trouble going from a bright to a dark room, and vice versa, or they may be confused by patterns or complex prints on wallpaper, furniture, or draperies.

The following suggestions can enable you to help a person see the best he or she can and prevent vision-related accidents.

- Create contrast where the potential for injury exists. Isaac always stumbled on the bottom step up to the second floor. Both the floor and the steps are of similar color wood, so Mariette painted a white strip across the bottom step. Other places that may need contrasting color are baseboards, around the edges and bottom of the bathtub and sink (use waterproof tape), banisters, and handrails.

- If individuals are disturbed by bright or complicated patterns on furniture or wall coverings, cover the furniture with plain sheets or towels rather than undergoing the expense of reupholstering them. Restrict access to rooms that have such patterns on the walls, and replace offending draperies with solid colors or textures.

- Provide enough light in rooms, hallways, and stairways. Leave a light on at night.

- Individuals who wear glasses will be less likely to lose them if the glasses are on a chain. Also keep a spare pair and the prescription handy in case the glasses are lost or broken.

- Contact lenses may become a problem. Have glasses made before the individual loses the ability to tend to the lenses properly.

It is important to distinguish between a vision problem and a disorder known as *agnosia*, which means "not to know." People with agnosia may have good vision, but their brain cannot properly process what they see. They may walk into a hole or a wall because their mind does not perceive those things as what they really are. "My wife looks right at me and says, 'Where is Curt? I can't find my husband. Please help me.' I tell her I'm Curt, but she says, 'No, you're not. I know my husband.' So she hasn't forgotten she has a husband. She just can't put together what she sees with whom she thinks she sees."

If you suspect the person may have developed a vision problem or agnosia, schedule an appointment for a complete eye exam. If the eye exam shows good vision, contact your physician so that the person may undergo further testing.

Hearing Problems

Imagine not knowing where you were or how you got there, and then discovering that you can't hear or understand what's being said. This is similar to what some people with Alzheimer's experience. "I can't tell if my father can't hear me or if he doesn't understand what I'm saying to him," said Libby. "He never had trouble hearing before, but he hasn't had his hearing checked in years. Is it Alzheimer's or age that's causing the problem?"

Suspected hearing loss should not be dismissed casually. An examination by an audiologist and a physician can usually detect the difference between an inability to understand and actual hearing loss; some individuals may have both conditions. Once the problem has been identified, appropriate action can be taken. "Our physician and the audiologist found that my father does have some hearing loss," said Libby, "but part of his problem is also that he can't process what people say to him. They suggested I try a hearing aid and see if he responds any better."

Libby bought a hearing aid with the understanding that she could bring it back if her father could not adjust to it. This is a good approach. Hearing aids augment background noise, and unless wearers are capable of adjusting the hearing aid to reduce such noise, they may become confused and agitated. In such cases no hearing aid may be a better alternative.

Whether or not individuals wear a hearing aid, the following suggestions may help improve their ability to attend to what they can hear:

• Speak in a low-pitched voice. High-pitched sounds are harder to hear and understand.
• Face the person when speaking and allow him or her to see your lips to increase understanding.
• Reduce the amount of background noise in the environment. Keep the radio on low. Avoid running loud appliances and "noise makers," such as a radio and television, simultaneously.
• Identify sounds and point out where they are com-

ing from. Say, "The robins are singing outside the kitchen window." "The dog is barking in the yard."

Dental Problems

Regular dental checkups as well as at-home monitoring are a must for people with Alzheimer's. Dentures and partial plates that are ill fitting may go unnoticed until an infection sets in or eating and nutrition problems occur. Carter assumed his wife was taking care of her teeth, as she always had. "I guess I should have paid more attention," he said. "Lena brushes her teeth fairly regularly, and I let her yearly checkup go by. When I noticed her cheek was swollen, I looked in her mouth and saw an abscess. I immediately called the dentist."

Although you may have a dentist you've gone to for many years, if he or she is not accustomed to working on people with Alzheimer's, consider finding one who is. If the person will not cooperate, the dentist may suggest giving a general anesthetic. Ask for an explanation of the risks versus the need for care before accepting the recommendation. Lena's dentist recommended giving her a general anesthetic because her tooth was infected and she was extremely restless in the dentist chair. Carter concurred and asked the dentist to examine and clean Lena's teeth at the same time. Carter also stayed with his wife throughout the entire procedure.

OTHER MEDICAL CONDITIONS

It is beyond the scope of this book to cover all preexisting or concurrent medical conditions the person with

Alzheimer's may have in addition to the disease itself. However, two conditions—hypertension and diabetes—are very common among the elderly, and the person you're caring for may have either or both of these treatable conditions. If so, you will need to ensure that medications are taken regularly and that they do not interfere with other medications the person may be taking. Both of these conditions are amenable to lifestyle changes such as following a healthful diet (see the next chapter) and getting regular exercise (see chapter 8). These modifications can be made early in the disease and may reduce the chances of drug interactions.

Hypertension

Various classes of drugs may be used to treat hypertension. Diuretics, which are discussed in the section on edema (pages 115–116), may also be prescribed for hypertension. Other drugs include beta-blockers, calcium channel blockers, and ACE inhibitors.

Beta-blockers

Beta-blockers, such as Sectral, Tenormin, and Inderal, are used to lower blood pressure, as well as to treat heart disease. They may be prescribed along with a low-dose diuretic. Side effects may include fatigue, dizziness, confusion, depression, nausea, diarrhea, and edema.

If the person you are caring for has any of these symptoms and he or she (or you, on his or her behalf) decides to stop taking the drug, contact your physician immediately. Beta-blockers should not be stopped suddenly. The physician will explain how to cut the dosage gradually.

Calcium Channel Blockers

Calcium channel blockers, such as Cardizem and Cardene, are members of another class of drugs that help lower blood pressure. Possible side effects of these drugs include dizziness, headache, constipation, edema, rash, or change in heart rate or rhythm.

ACE Inhibitors

Angiotensin converting enzyme (ACE) inhibitors, yet another group of medications to lower blood pressure, include drugs such as Capoten, Vasotec, and Prinivil.

These drugs are sometimes given to individuals who have both hypertension and diabetes, but they are usually avoided in people with kidney disease. Side effects may include rash, dizziness, change in heart rate, chest pain, headache, hacking cough, and metallic taste.

Diabetes

If the person you are caring for has diabetes, you may need to learn how to administer the daily insulin injections and monitor blood sugar levels. A counselor from the American Diabetes Association can show you how, or you can ask for help from your physician or a nurse.

The person you are caring for may require oral hypoglycemic pills. If you are caring for someone who takes this medication, alert your physician if he or she also is taking any of the following drugs, which can cause variations in blood sugar levels: aspirin, diuretics, estrogen, niacin, Adrenalin, decongestants that contain epinephrine or ephedrine, cough remedies, nasal sprays that contain phenylephrine, or over-the-counter drugs that contain caffeine.

HOSPITALIZATION

Sometimes a person with Alzheimer's needs to be hospitalized for other medical conditions. This can be very stressful for both of you. Many people with Alzheimer's become combative or abusive when they are admitted to the hospital. "My husband had to go into the hospital when he fell and broke his hip," said Carmela. "Edwin is very confused most of the time, and I worried that the strange environment would make it worse. And it did. He yelled and tried to hit the nurses. I was there as much as I could be, but he didn't always know me."

The sudden shift in environment, people, and activities throws people with Alzheimer's into a state of confusion. Be assured that this heightened level of confusion usually subsides once they return home. While in the hospital, however, it may be necessary to sedate or restrain them for a short time. "When Edwin woke up, he immediately tried to remove his intravenous tubes. I thought the nurses were going to tie him down, but they said they would try putting mittens on him first. The mittens discouraged him, and he gave up on the tubes."

Generally the least amount of restraint required, the better. Restraints can be frightening and can cause some individuals to become more agitated and combative. You cannot stop the person you are caring for from being upset, but you can make his or her time in the hospital as comfortable as possible and, in the process, make your time easier too. Following are some suggestions:

• Before admission, discuss the person's condition and behavior with the physician. Ask if outpatient treatment is an option.

- Let the nursing staff know what the person can and cannot do (toileting habits, feeding, grooming). Write down the person's favorite foods and the names of people he or she may ask for.
- Bring items to the hospital that the person can feel comforted by, such as photographs, stuffed animals, or familiar clothing.
- Ask a family member or friend to stay with the individual when you are not able to be there. "We visited Edwin in shifts," explained Carmela. "My sister went in the morning and stayed until lunch. I fed him lunch and stayed through dinner. Then the grandchildren came at night."

Unfortunately over time the person you're caring for is likely to experience an increasing number of medical problems as the disease progresses. This is why ultimately most caregivers are forced to consider alternative living situations for the person (see chapter 9). However, if the course of the disease is slow, such problems may take years to manifest themselves. In the meantime there is much you can do to ensure that the person experiences the best possible quality of life from day to day, including making sure the person enjoys proper nutrition, exercise, social activity, and lowered stress levels—all of which are important for you as well. These topics will be covered in detail in the following chapters.

SEVEN

Mealtimes and Nutrition

"Peter picked up his fork and put it down without eating anything. I thought he wasn't hungry. Then he put his hands into the mashed potatoes and ate them off his fingers. I was stunned! Then I realized that he had forgotten how to use the fork. So I showed him how to use it, and for a few days, he imitated me—and then forgot again. Now I just give him food he can eat with his hands, such as sandwiches or fruit. Why frustrate him—and myself—any further? The disease is taking its toll. The man I married is becoming more and more helpless. I'm terribly sad, but I'm adapting, doing what I can to help him while he can still be at home. And I tell myself, 'At least he's still able to eat.' I know that once he can no longer feed himself, I won't be able to help for long."

—Mary

Poor eating behaviors often mean more than having to clean up spilled soup or coaxing a person to eat. Some people with Alzheimer's disease want to eat everything in sight; others refuse to eat at all. Some people focus on one or two foods and will ignore your attempts to get them to eat anything else. Others will insist they are hungry even though they have just finished a meal. As Valerie noted, "Bob would eat all day if I let him. I have to hide food from him. After he finishes dinner, he says, 'I'm hungry. I want to eat.' It doesn't help to tell him he just ate."

As memory and physical functioning deteriorate, problems with eating increase, resulting in poor nutritional intake. Inadequate consumption of calories, protein, vitamins, and other essential elements can cause malnutrition, weight loss, bowel irregularities, and other medical problems.

In this chapter we'll review how to overcome many of the roadblocks that may stand in the way of the person's ability to eat appropriately, enjoy food, and reap the benefits of good nutrition. We'll also cover the basics of sound nutrition and offer suggestions for planning meals that are healthful and pleasing.

PROBLEM EATING BEHAVIOR

Physical problems that limit the person's ability to use eating utensils or to chew and swallow food, as well as emotional upset, depression, distractions in the environment, and biochemical disorders in the brain are among the many factors that may interfere with appetite and rob mealtime of its pleasure.

Inadequate Food Intake

If the person you're caring for appears to have lost his or her appetite or resists eating, you will need to determine the reason before you can take appropriate steps. Consider the following possibilities:

- Ill-fitting dentures or other dental problems may make eating painful. Check the person's mouth for sores, infections, or other signs that dentures or partial plates are not fitted properly. Schedule a dental examination if you suspect a problem.
- People who are anxious, confused, or distracted may walk away from their meal or fidget and not eat. Are there noises, odors, or other distractions in the room that may be bothering them? Try to keep the environment as calm as possible.
- Physical problems such as constipation, dry mouth, or stomach upset, and medical conditions such as diabetes, colitis, heart problems, and ulcers may decrease appetite. A physical examination may be needed to determine whether these problems are at the root of poor eating behavior.
- People with vision problems may not see food clearly, leading to lack of recognition of the food, or confusion. Note whether they have trouble seeing other objects that are at close range. If so, it may be helpful to have the person wear glasses at mealtime (or change a current prescription that is no longer appropriate).
- Medications such as NSAIDs or antidepressants may have the side effect of decreasing appetite. Consult with your physician if you suspect this may be the reason the person is not eating.
- The person may have forgotten how to use the utensils or find they are too hard to manipulate. To test this theory, place a utensil in the person's hand, and you do the same. Pick up some food on your utensil and see if the person mimics you. If not, guide his or her utensil to pick up food. While raising your food to your mouth, guide the person's utensil to his or her mouth. After this

demonstration the person may continue to feed himself or herself. You may have to repeat this process at every meal, however.

- Some people can no longer recognize what food is. This is a condition known as agnosia, in which the brain does not correctly process what the eyes see (see chapter 6). Serve their favorite foods to see if they refuse them as well.

Increased Appetite

Sometimes the appetite mechanism in the brain is damaged, causing individuals who have just eaten to insist they are still hungry. "I can never leave food out, or Carmine will eat it. He follows me around and says, 'Hungry, hungry' even when he's just eaten," says Sophie. "Sometimes I feel like I'm being mean if I don't give him something. But even when I do, he's back ten minutes later saying he's hungry again."

Reminding the person that he or she has just eaten will not mean anything. Instead try these approaches:

- Keep your kitchen cabinets and refrigerator locked.
- Remove any form of food—including candy and gum—from sight (candy dishes, kitchen counter, cookie jars, and so forth).
- Feed the person five or six small meals a day, or dispense nutritious snacks throughout the day instead of three large meals. If weight gain begins to be a problem, consult with your physician or nutritionist.

Disruptive Behavior

Some eating problems involve more than reluctance or refusal to eat. "My husband can throw a mean bowl of cereal," said Tammy. "Sid's not always that disruptive, but I don't take any chances. I use plastic bowls and plates, plastic drinking cups with lids, a vinyl tablecloth —whatever won't break and I can clean up easily. I don't use plastic spoons or forks because they can break, and Sid could hurt himself."

Some individuals will do everything with their food except eat it: throw it, spit it out, or play with it. Others will eat things they shouldn't, such as coins or stones. Check to see whether some "logical" reason is causing the person to spit or throw food: The food is unfamiliar, it's too hot or cold, he or she doesn't like the smell, is upset by something in the surroundings, or can't manipulate the utensils.

If the person is disruptive despite attempts to make food more acceptable, stop the meal by either removing the food or taking the person for a short walk. Try to resume the meal when he or she is calmer.

To minimize the consequences of these behaviors, try the following:

• Use bowls instead of plates, paper or plastic instead of ceramic or china.
• To prevent dishes from being thrown, consider purchasing plates, cups, and bowls with suction cups from medical supply houses.
• Avoid spills by using cups with lids and bendable straws.

- Place a plastic placemat under the person's plate and a plastic dropcloth on the floor to make cleanup easier.
- Keep bottles of ketchup, mustard, salad dressing, soy sauce, and other condiments off the dining room table and out of reach. "When I wasn't looking, my sister grabbed a bottle of oil off the kitchen table and drank half of it before I caught her," said Karla. "She simply doesn't recognize what she should and should not eat."
- For your own sake minimize messiness. "Sometimes Mark drops his spoon and puts his hands into his food. Then he smears it on his clothes. Getting him to wear a bib was impossible, and I can understand how that probably made him feel. Now I have designated 'food shirts.' He wears an oversized shirt over his regular clothes when he eats. It has stains that will never come out, but who cares? I just throw it into the wash."

PROBLEMS WITH CHEWING, SWALLOWING, OR DROOLING

As the disease progresses, some individuals have trouble chewing and swallowing. They may forget to chew at all and try to swallow their food whole. If they have lost muscle strength or coordination, poor posture may cause them to choke. Drooling, another common symptom of Alzheimer's, may be the result of weakened muscles, medications, or food being held in the mouth and not swallowed.

The following suggestions can help you minimize problems and maximize nutritional intake for these individuals:

- Make sure dentures and partial plates fit properly.
- Serve foods that require little or no chewing: cottage cheese, soups, juices, yogurt, puddings, tofu, milk shakes, mashed potatoes, oatmeal, applesauce, and scrambled eggs. You can use a food processor or food grinder to make pureed fruits, vegetables, and meats. Ask your physician or nutritionist for ideas on how to maintain a balanced diet using soft foods.
- The mouth loses sensation in some people with Alzheimer's. Gently move their chin to remind them to chew. Lightly stroke their throat to remind them to swallow.
- Avoid foods that contain two textures—for example, cereal and milk or chunky soups—because the individual may not know whether to chew or swallow and may end up choking.
- Avoid baby foods if possible. These can be demoralizing to people with Alzheimer's.
- Watch the person's posture and encourage him or her to sit up straight with the head slightly forward.
- When feeding a person who is bedridden, encourage him or her to maintain as vertical a position as possible. Use a bed tray and protect the person and the surrounding bedclothes with washable coverings. Use an oversized spoon filled half or two-thirds with food. Apply slight pressure on the bottom lip to encourage the person to open his or her mouth, followed by the reminder "Now swallow."
- Learn the Heimlich maneuver in order to help the person if choking occurs. If the person can cough, speak, or breathe, do not interfere. If he or she cannot cough, speak, or breathe, you must help. If the person is sitting or standing, stand behind the person with your arms

around the waist. Make a fist and place it in the middle of the person's abdomen, below the ribs. Grab your fist with the other hand and pull hard and quickly back and upward four or five times. This should force air up through the throat and cause food to come flying out.

If the person is lying down, turn him or her faceup. Kneel next to the person's legs and put the heel of your hand on the abdomen, below the ribs and slightly above the navel. Place your other hand on top of the first, and make four or five forceful thrusts downward and forward toward the person's head. Check the person's mouth for an obstruction and remove it.

SUCCESSFUL MEALTIMES

Simplicity and patience are key ingredients for successful mealtimes. Each eating experience should be as tension-free as possible for both of you. Here are some ways to achieve this:

• Consider what the individual's eating patterns and preferences used to be, such as favorite foods and routine eating times, and continue them. "My mother never ate lunch. She always had a glass of juice when she got up and then a full breakfast around ten o'clock, after she did some of her housework," said Rhoda. "Then she'd have dinner on the table at five. That was her routine for thirty years. Trying to get her to eat three meals a day was impossible, and really not practical when I think about it. Why should I force her to change? When I switched to her old routine, she stopped fighting me at mealtimes. It was a relief for both of us."

- Strive for a relaxed atmosphere. Play classical music in the background. Avoid distractions such as television or loud noises. If necessary, take the phone off the hook during meals.
- Establish a routine and stick to it. Serve meals at the same time and place daily, using the same place settings (dishes, tablecloth, placemats, utensils). Familiarity reduces confusion.
- Test foods to make sure they are not too hot or too cold. Many people with Alzheimer's lose some of their ability to sense temperatures accurately.
- Eating is a highly social event in our society. Don't let the person you're caring for eat alone. Ask family members and friends to visit for a meal. Talk with the person you're caring for, maintain eye contact, and show by your expression that you are enjoying your food. The person may follow your lead.
- If having two or three types of food on the plate is causing confusion, serve only one item at a time.
- Serve the meal ready to eat. For example, have the food already cut, the vegetables buttered, and the drinks poured.
- People who have trouble using utensils can be given finger foods, such as cheese and crackers, vegetable crudités, chicken nuggets, fish sticks, pizza, sandwiches, and grapes and other fruit cut into bite-sized pieces. Broth and cream soups can be put into mugs instead of bowls. Individuals with limited dexterity may find it easier—and less dangerous—to use a spoon than a fork. Adaptive utensils usually aren't necessary, and people with Alzheimer's often have difficulty learning to use them.
- Allow the individual plenty of time to finish the

meal. "It takes Isabel about an hour to get through dinner," said Dodge. "She can still feed herself pretty well, but she needs reminders to keep going. If I get up and try to do the dishes or something else before she's done, she refuses to eat. So I've learned to be patient and not hurry her along. I sit with her, do a crossword puzzle, and keep reminding her to eat."

MAINTAINING GOOD NUTRITION

Good nutrition is important to you as well as to the person you're caring for. If you don't eat well, you may become more tense and irritable, and your resistance will be lowered. A balanced diet will help both of you avoid other illnesses and cope with the stress of chronic illness. Be aware that there is no scientific evidence that nutrition helps any aspect of Alzheimer's disease or that a special diet can improve memory. However, there is no question that following a balanced daily diet can help both of you maintain good health and well-being, and probably lessen stress and fatigue.

On the other hand poor eating habits can eventually result in problems such as malnutrition, constipation, diarrhea, fatigue, listlessness, and dental problems, to name a few. All can be especially serious in people with Alzheimer's because of their deteriorating mental and physical condition.

Malnutrition

When the doctor told Albert that his wife, Janice, was malnourished, he was shocked. "Malnutrition! It sounded like I was starving her. The doctor told me he realized it was difficult to get her to eat, and it is. I have to spoon-feed her, and often it takes an hour to get through one bowl of soup. The doctor told me to give Janice a liquid supplement between meals to help build up her strength and prevent any serious illness. She seems to like the supplements, and she can take them through a straw."

Weight alone is not a good indication of whether someone is malnourished. Even overweight people can be malnourished. Brad eats three times a day, but as his wife said, "It's all junk. The only things he likes are french fries, potato chips, pork rinds—anything fried or fatty. I try disguising vegetables such as eggplant and squash by breading and frying them, but I know that's not really good for him either. If I don't give him what he wants, he won't eat at all."

Eating too much "junk" food, especially those foods high in fat or sugar (candy, ice cream, cake, cookies), can result in too many calories being consumed but not enough essential elements. In some cases it may be necessary to enrich the individual's diet with a vitamin, mineral, or protein supplement.

Other Consequences

Constipation is often related to diet and can be caused by inadequate intake of fiber and fluids. Good sources of fiber include vegetables and fruits (mash or steam them if chewing and swallowing are a problem), whole-grain cereals and breads (add bran to cold and hot cereals), and beans and lentils (pureed legumes, added to broth and finely chopped vegetables makes a good soup). Eight glasses of juice or water daily will help prevent not only constipation but also dehydration, which can be a problem in people who take diuretics.

Insufficient intake of calories and essential nutrients compound the physical deterioration experienced by people with Alzheimer's. Individuals who eat a large amount of sugar may experience mood and behavior swings—periods of increased activity soon after they eat the sweets followed by depression, listlessness, and fatigue.

If the person you are caring for also suffers from diabetes, hypertension, or a heart condition, these conditions may worsen if the proper diet is not followed. Every effort should be made to ensure that a healthful diet —low in fat and cholesterol, moderate in calories—is followed. The person should have periodic lab tests to ensure that improper diet is not adversely affecting glucose or cholesterol levels.

MENU PLANNING

According to the U.S. Department of Agriculture, a balanced daily diet consists of six to eleven servings of cereal, pasta, rice, and bread; two to three of yogurt, cheese, and milk; two to three of meat, poultry, fish, eggs, cheese, dried beans, peas, or nuts; three to five of vegetables; two to four of fruit. In reality, however, many caregivers have trouble meeting these goals, both for themselves and for the person for whom they're caring. Rather than worrying about numbers of servings of food per day, try keeping the following basic guidelines in mind. They are approved by major health organizations such as the American Heart Association and the American Dietetic Association.

Increase Variety

Encourage the person you are caring for to eat foods from all food groups, with special emphasis on grains, fruit, and vegetables, as well as low-fat milk and cheese products and low-fat fish, meat, and poultry.

Increase Fiber

Foods in their natural state such as fruits, vegetables, beans, peas, nuts, and whole-grain breads and cereals contain complex carbohydrates and fiber, and are generally more healthful than refined foods such as most bakery products and candy.

Fiber helps relieve constipation and is associated with reduced risk of heart disease and certain cancers. Fiber also promotes a feeling of fullness, which can help if the patient is overweight and needs to curb his or her appetite.

Fiber supplements are not recommended unless prescribed by a physician.

Avoid Excess Fat

Too much saturated fat and cholesterol in the diet may contribute to the development of heart disease and stroke. To reduce excess fat in the diet:

- Reduce consumption of saturated fats from animal products (beef, pork, lamb, veal, butter, cream, cheese) by trimming fat from meat, removing skin from poultry, and substituting low- or nonfat dairy products for those made with whole milk. Also avoid saturated vegetable fats—cocoa butter, palm oil, coconut oil—which are often found in bakery items, candies, fried foods, and nondairy milk and cream substitute.

• Reduce consumption of hydrogenated fats, contained in margarine, some brands of peanut butter, and a wide variety of processed foods, such as crackers and cookies (check ingredient labels when shopping).

• Limit intake of organ meats (liver, sweetbreads), which are very high in fat and cholesterol.

• Broil, boil, bake, or steam foods instead of frying. Use a spray-on vegetable oil when sautéing.

• Read labels to determine the percentage of fat in foods. Try to use products that have less than 30 percent of calories from fat.

Avoid Excess Cholesterol

Cholesterol intake should be less than 300 milligrams per day (one egg yolk contains about 213 milligrams of cholesterol—use egg substitutes in baking and don't serve more than three eggs per week). By replacing much of your meat and poultry meals with recipes that emphasize pastas (without creamy sauces), whole grains, vegetables, and fruits, cholesterol (and fat) intake will be dramatically lowered.

Avoid Excess Sugar

Sugar is a source of "empty" calories, since it provides no nutrients. To reduce the amount of sugar in the diet:

- Use less of all sugars, including white, brown, and raw sugars, honey, and syrups. None of these forms of pure sugar is significantly better for you than any other.
- Substitute fresh fruit or canned fruit in its own juice or water for sugary foods such as candy, soft drinks, cake, and cookies.
- Watch for hidden sugar. When reading labels, be aware that *sucrose, glucose, dextrose, lactose, fructose, maltose, corn syrup,* and *corn sweetener* are all words that mean sugar. If any of these are among the first ingredients listed on the label, then the product contains a large amount of sugar.

Avoid Excess Sodium

Excess salt, either from the salt shaker or in foods naturally high in salt, increases the risk of hypertension, which is a major factor in heart disease and stroke.

To limit the amount of salt in the diet:

- Add little or no salt to food when cooking.
- Be aware that salt hides under several names. When reading food labels, the word *sodium* means an item contains salt. Disodium phosphate, monosodium glutamate, sodium chloride, and sodium nitrate are a few of the ingredients that are actually various types of salt compounds.
- Avoid foods with a high salt or sodium content, such as bacon, canned soups and gravies, canned vegetables, potato chips, pretzels, salted nuts, cheese, prepackaged dinners, and many bakery desserts.
- Be aware that many food flavorings are high in salt. Bouillon cubes, chili sauce, garlic salt, onion salt, meat

tenderizers, pickles, soy sauce, ketchup, and Worcestershire sauce all have a high sodium content (though many of these products are now available in low-salt versions).

Limit Alcohol

Alcoholic beverages, like sugar, are high in calories and low in nutritional value. In addition, alcohol—even in moderate quantities—may contribute to the physical and mental deterioration of the person with Alzheimer's and lead to accidents, with potentially disastrous consequences.

Limit Caffeine

Beverages with a high caffeine content, such as coffee, tea, and cola drinks, should be consumed in moderation. Caffeine has a stimulating effect on the nervous system, which may cause the person to become jittery or lightheaded. Decaffeinated beverages are rarely caffeine-free, and if consumed in sufficient quantity, even these may cause a caffeine reaction. Instead substitute more healthful liquids, such as water or fruit juice.

Maintain Ideal Weight

Being overweight increases the risk of a number of diseases, including heart disease, hypertension, and diabetes —all of which contribute to the risk of heart attack or stroke. Excess weight also decreases mobility and interferes with daily activities.

TIPS FOR IMPROVING NUTRITIONAL INTAKE

Although it is often difficult to meet all the accepted requirements for a balanced diet, it is important to keep trying. Try the following suggestions for improving the nutritional intake of the person you're caring for. Some of these strategies will work for you; others will not. Some may work one day and not the next. All of them have been successful at some point for many people.

- Serve a large meal at breakfast or lunch rather than at dinner. Some people with Alzheimer's have a bigger appetite in the morning than at night.
- If individuals refuse to eat more than a few bites before becoming distracted or getting up from the table, try presenting nutritious snacks or small meals several times a day to ensure adequate nutrition. Some handy snack items are grapes, raisins, yogurt, apple and orange slices, bananas, milk shakes, vegetable sticks (you may want to steam carrots, celery, peppers, and broccoli for easier chewing), cheese, and whole-grain crackers and breadsticks.
- Serve a cup of broth or a glass of juice before a meal to stimulate the appetite.
- Increase the nutritional value of foods the person is eating already: Stir wheat germ into cereal or oatmeal; whip an egg or egg substitute into a milk shake; add sesame seeds, crushed nuts, or fresh fruit to ice cream; make healthful cookies or muffins using bran, raisins, and wheat germ; puree vegetables and add them to canned soups or, if you have time, make your own soup; blend fresh fruit (apples, pears, bananas, strawberries) with honey for dessert.

As noted earlier, if the individual is not getting enough calories or is not following a balanced diet regardless of your best efforts, your physician may suggest a vitamin supplement. If he or she recommends a liquid food supplement, ask how to make your own, as these supplements are often expensive.

MEAL-PREPARATION TIPS

Preparing nutritious meals day in and day out can be a tiring task on top of everything else you must do. For some caregivers such as Zoran, cooking is a new experience—making the job doubly difficult.

"My wife always did all the cooking," said Zoran. "I hate to depend on TV dinners, so I bought a cookbook full of easy, one-step meals. Now I make do with the few things I know how to make well."

Fortunately there are several ways to make sure both you and the person you care for enjoy good meals with a minimum of effort:

• Meals on Wheels will deliver a hot meal to your home. Many community centers and religious organizations also offer lunch programs at a minimal cost. Both of these options relieve you of preparing at least one meal a day. Contact your social worker, county Office of Aging, or church, or look under "Social Services Organizations" in the Yellow Pages. Also see chapter 12.

• Utilize restaurant takeout and home-delivery services; however, be careful to order foods that are relatively low in fat and moderate in calories, such as grilled fish or poultry and steamed vegetables or baked potatoes.

- Take cooking classes. Many schools, community centers, and other organizations offer adult-education cooking classes that focus on easy-to-prepare meals.

Shopping Tips

- Make a shopping list that includes foods the person enjoys.
- Buy a mixture of green leafy vegetables (spinach, mustard or collard greens, kale), cruciferous vegetables (broccoli, brussels sprouts), and yellow vegetables (squash, pumpkin, peppers) to be eaten in salads or steamed as side dishes.
- Buy a variety of fruits (apples, pears, grapes, oranges, bananas). Some can be eaten steamed or cooked for breakfast, snacks, and dessert.
- Don't forget grains, cereals, breads, pasta, rice, potatoes, and other foods high in complex carbohydrates to form the foundation of your meals.
- Try legumes, which are high in protein and low in fat: black, garbanzo, lima, mung, kidney, and pinto beans; black-eyed, yellow, and green peas; lentils and nuts and seeds.
- Stick with low-fat sources of animal protein—chicken breast without skin, fish, trimmed beef, lean pork.

- Buy low or nonfat dairy products, including milk, yogurt, and various types of reduced-fat cheeses.
- Avoid prepared foods from the deli counter (potato salad, cole slaw, tuna or chicken salad) since these are generally loaded with oil and mayonnaise.
- Carefully check the labels of frozen dinners. In addition to being expensive, many are high in salt and preservatives and lack sufficient vitamins, fiber, or other essential nutrients.

A registered dietitian or other health professional knowledgeable in nutrition can assist you in planning appropriate special diets (i.e., weight-loss, diabetic) that also provide adequate nutrition for overall good health. At the same time you can help the person you're caring for maintain health and enjoy a better quality of life through regular physical activity and socializing. The next chapter will tell you how.

EIGHT

Exercise, Socializing, and Other Activities

"Sara can't dress herself anymore, and she needs help when she eats, but she still takes a walk every day. Of course I go with her; we walk around the park. Actually it's a relaxing time for me too."

—Abe

"It's the strangest thing. My wife doesn't know me most of the time, and she can't remember where the bathroom is, but she can still sit down and play the piano as if nothing were wrong with her. And she loves to sing the old songs. We sing them together. It's the only time I feel there's still a connection between us."

—Drew

Physical activity, socializing, and recreation are essential for everyone, including people with Alzheimer's. Although none of these activities can halt the progression of the disease, they can enrich the lives of those with the disease and ease the burden of care for caregivers. They can also facilitate meaningful interaction between caregivers and the people in their care.

In this chapter we'll look at how you can help make

exercise, socializing, and recreational activities an enriching part of the lives of the person you're caring for, and the benefits you can both reap from these activities.

Be sure both of you consult your physician before starting an exercise program. Medications, plus any pre-existing conditions—cardiovascular problems, stroke, arthritis—may affect the type or amount of exercise that can be undertaken safely.

EXERCISE HAS MANY BENEFITS

Too often exercise is viewed only as a way of losing weight or helping to stay in shape. While those are some of the benefits, exercise has many other advantages, especially for people with Alzheimer's. "Alistair is in a wheelchair. But we go for a walk every day," said his wife, Robyn. "Now he sleeps so much better." Other advantages include the following:

- Regular activity is an effective outlet for nervousness, anxiety, and tension; thus people with Alzheimer's who are physically active may not fidget and pace as much as they would otherwise.
- Night wanderers who exercise tend to wander less.
- Exercise can relieve constipation and stimulate the appetite in poor eaters.
- Some professionals believe the deterioration of motor functioning may be slowed in individuals who exercise.
- Exercise allows caregivers and the person in their care to interact on a different, and hopefully fun, level.

Selecting Appropriate Exercises

Exercise can be approached in several ways, depending on the capabilities of the person with Alzheimer's and the setting in which exercise is performed. It's better to exercise a little every day than attempting a long session once or twice a week.

The first consideration is ability: Individuals who are ambulatory and flexible obviously have more options than those with impaired functioning, but even people in wheelchairs and those confined can and should exercise.

The second consideration is setting: Where can he or she—and you too—exercise? In the house, the yard, a neighborhood park, a community center—or a combination of these facilities? Many adult-day-care centers (see chapter 9) offer recreational activities specifically for people with Alzheimer's disease.

"Until my husband became so disoriented and confused that I couldn't be sure of his behavior, we went to the YMCA every morning and used the exercise equipment," said Helen. *"Now I take him to adult day care, where they offer calisthenics every day. We still take a short walk in the evening before dinner too."*

The third consideration is preference. Try to choose activities you both enjoy, or ones that are similar to the types of activities the person with Alzheimer's used to engage in prior to becoming ill.

Walking is of course an excellent exercise that is suitable for most people. Pace and distance will depend on the individual's physical and mental condition. Some people may feel less confused if you take the same route every time.

If the weather is inclement, or if you do not live in an area that is safe to walk in, drive to an enclosed mall and walk there. Many malls also have early-morning walking programs so that people can stroll before the stores open. This can be helpful for disoriented individuals, who may be upset by crowds.

Calisthenics can be done at home or at a day-care or recreational center. Many people with Alzheimer's like to mimic other people's movements, and enjoy exercising in groups.

During exercise sessions in the home it may be helpful to do movements to music of your choice; you may also consider purchasing a video with easy calisthenics. Hold on to the back of a chair to help maintain balance.

Dancing is another option, as Kenneth discovered. "The senior center has ballroom and free-form dance sessions every afternoon. Lucy and I were attending the ballroom sessions, but they became a little too difficult for her, so now she does free-form dance. She loves it. I bought some tapes for home so that she can dance on the weekends too."

People who formerly played golf or tennis can frequently continue these activities through the early stage of Alzheimer's. As their abilities decline, golfers may still enjoy the driving range or putting, and tennis players may practice hitting balls against a wall. Even cyclists may be able to keep up this activity. Jackson used to ride his bike twenty or thirty miles several times a week. When it was no longer safe for him to go out on the road, his son bought him a stationary bike. "I purchased the low-slung model. The seat is close to the floor, so

Dad's legs are out in front while he pedals," says his son. "That way he can't fall off and hurt himself."

Wheelchair Exercises

Exercises for a person confined to a wheelchair are designed to increase circulation and help maintain some flexibility and muscle strength.

Many people with Alzheimer's who are confined to a wheelchair are in the moderate-to-severe stages of disease. They often need to be prompted through each movement; some may be able to mimic your actions. Help the person try the following, increasing or decreasing the number of repetitions depending upon his or her ability:

- Slowly rotate the head clockwise and counterclockwise. Bend the head down toward the chest, then lift the head back toward the spine. Do each movement three times.
- Stretch the arms overhead and reach the fingers out as far as they will go. Hold for several seconds and then return the arms to the sides. Repeat four times.
- Stretch arms straight in front. Open and close the hands several times. Return the arms to the sides and repeat the sequence four times.
- Shrug, then rotate the shoulders forward and backward. Repeat three times.
- Lift the right knee; rotate the foot three times to the right and to the left. Place the foot back down. Repeat with the left leg.
- Lift the right leg up as high as you comfortably can, hold for two to three seconds, then return it to the leg

rest or floor. Do the same with the left leg. Repeat eight to ten times.

• Sit as straight as possible while remaining comfortable. Take a deep breath. Lift the arms overhead while inhaling, and slowly lower them while exhaling. Repeat five times.

Exercising in Bed

People who are confined to bed need to stretch their muscles and joints to avoid atrophy (muscle wasting) and contracture (shortening of the tendons and ligaments). This latter condition can be very painful and may cause individuals to move into a permanent fetal position.

These exercises begin with the person lying on his or her back. Each exercise should be done first with one leg, then with the other. You will probably have to assist the person through each movement.

• Keeping the knee slightly bent, lift the leg up as far as it will go comfortably. Hold for two to three seconds, then slowly lower it.

• Lift the leg, rotate the foot to the right and then to the left. Lower the leg.

• Lift the leg, bend the knee and bring the knee toward the chest. Hold for two seconds. Straighten the leg and lower it slowly.

• Stretch both arms up toward the ceiling (if the person is weak, do one arm at a time). Rotate the arms in the sockets. Flex the fingers and rotate the wrists. Return the arms to the sides.

• Lift the head off the pillow, hold for several seconds,

and return it to the pillow. Turn the head to the right and left several times.

- Take a deep breath. Lift the arms overhead, inhaling, and slowly down while exhaling. Repeat three times.

General Tips for Exercising Regularly

- Establish a routine and stick with it. Structure helps the person with Alzheimer's feel more oriented and helps ensure that you will do the exercises regularly.
- Time exercise to your advantage. A late-afternoon or early-evening activity may be best for people who have trouble sleeping. Those who are restless or agitated may benefit from split sessions: ten minutes of dancing in the morning, a short walk in the afternoon, and stretching exercises before retiring. These activities can be good tension relievers for you as well.
- Since people with Alzheimer's often enjoy mimicking, when exercising at home, demonstrate in front of the person; wait between each movement so that the person has time to imitate you.
- Incorporate exercise and stretching movements into daily activities. The walk to the mailbox may be short, but make it as brisk as possible. Show the person you're caring for how to do a slow stretch when putting on shoes and socks. Do gentle bending and stretching movements while watching television.
- People with Alzheimer's have a short attention span and are easily distracted, so keep exercise sessions short —ten to twenty minutes at most for such activities as calisthenics and dancing. You may be able to walk for longer periods if you keep the person interested by point-

ing out scenery or making frequent stops to look at sights along the way. "Glenn and I usually walk for an hour," said Christine. "We take the same route every day, past the florist, where we always stop to look at the flowers. Sometimes Glenn anticipates that stop, but other times it seems new to him. Then we go to the park and feed the squirrels. We walk every day if we can, but if the weather is bad and we stay home, I notice he's more restless."

• Be aware of the person's limitations. People who have balance or vision problems need to be watched closely during exercise. Stop exercising immediately if the person appears dizzy or confused.

A SOCIAL LIFE IS POSSIBLE

Ideally people with Alzheimer's should be encouraged to participate in the same social activities they enjoyed before becoming ill, making adjustments as the disease progresses. Some professionals believe continued socialization may help prolong the amount of time a person remains in the early stage of Alzheimer's. It is also likely to improve their mood and stave off depression. "My mother was a volunteer at the hospital for twenty years," said Tanya. "She has a lot of friends there. During the early stage of Alzheimer's she cut back on her time from twenty-five hours to fifteen. They let her work alongside another volunteer and do easy tasks, such as filling the water pitchers and collecting the menus. She sat with her friends at lunch. When she became too confused, she stopped working and moved in with my husband and me. But one or two volunteers still come once a week and bring lunch to Mom. She doesn't always remember who they are, but occasionally she responds to something they say. I believe these visits make her feel good, and they give me some relief."

Before planning social activities for the person with Alzheimer's, consider the following factors:

- Individuals who are in the early stages of the disease should be allowed to choose the activities they would like to participate in. Forcing them to do repetitive tasks or "busywork" can be demoralizing. Foster their need for independence. Once they can no longer make decisions, however, you will have to select and guide their activities for them.
- Encourage activities that are familiar and comfortable. Now is not the time to teach the person how to play checkers or bridge.
- Expect the unexpected. People with Alzheimer's may enjoy an activity one day and refuse to do it the next. Olive had joined the sing-along at the senior center every Monday and Friday for several weeks. "Then one Friday she just refused to go," said her sister, Victoria. "I tried again a week later and she still wasn't interested."
- Routinely monitor the person's ability to participate in the activity. Eventually his or her level of response will deteriorate; then it will be time to either simplify the activity, move on to another one, or stop. Victoria guessed that Olive couldn't remember the words to the songs and, frustrated, refused to join the group. To allow Olive to still enjoy the music, Victoria encouraged her to sit with other seniors who act as the "audience."

Types of Activities

For as long as possible, the social activities of people with Alzheimer's should include family gatherings and visits with friends, as well as participation in programs in the community.

Be aware, however, that large groups may be difficult to cope with, so have a quiet corner or room for the person to go to if stress becomes a problem. Grandchildren, for example, may be a great comfort, but too many at once may cause distress.

Keep family members and other visitors up-to-date on the person's condition so that they know what to expect in terms of interaction. Explain what the person may or may not be able to understand and that he or she may tire easily.

If visitors insist on bringing a gift, suggest food, a music or book cassette, or flowers. As the person with Alzheimer's becomes less able to hold a conversation, expect that many people may feel uneasy and therefore stay away. Their abandonment, although understandable, will be felt by the person with Alzheimer's as well as by you. This may be the time to look into the activities held at adult-day-care and senior-citizen centers.

For some men and women with Alzheimer's, work was the focus of social interaction, and declining abilities eventually exclude them from that environment. If their employer agrees, see whether they might go to the office part-time and do small tasks or attend meetings. Gilbert was vice president of a local bank when his failing memory made it necessary for him to retire after twenty-eight years with the organization. Gilbert's wife asked the bank president whether her husband might sit in on some of the staff meetings. He agreed, and Gilbert attends the weekly sessions.

An alternative to staying at one's job is to do volunteer work. This provides a service to the community and also builds the sense of self-worth of the person with Alzheimer's. Organizations often need help with routine mailings, sorting clothes, stacking books, handing out snacks, and other easy but necessary tasks.

Outings to public places, such as restaurants, concerts, the mall, theater, museums, church, and the park are encouraged as long as they are not stressful or disruptive for the person or for you. Keep visits short and sit near an exit in case you need to leave quickly. Choose times when there may be fewer people attending—for example, the earliest church service or four o'clock at a restaurant.

Contact with nature can be very comforting, especially for people who are confined indoors much of the time. A visit to a park or even sitting in the backyard, especially for those confined to a wheelchair, can be a pleasant diversion. Take along food for the birds or squirrels, or set up a bird feeder in the backyard. A picnic in the park may be an alternative to eating in a restaurant; an outdoor concert better than one in a hall.

Children and Pets

Some experts believe young children and pets are among the best companions for people with Alzheimer's. Both can give unquestioning affection and attention. If possible, arrange for young grandchildren or those of friends or neighbors to visit. You might make such visits a regular event. For example, Marlene invites two of the neighbors' children over every Monday afternoon to visit with her father, George. Both children are three years old, and their mothers visit with Marlene while George colors and draws with the two girls. "The girls think it's a party," said Marlene. "I have cookies and balloons for them, and the mothers bring juice. It gives us an hour or two to chat. My father's mood is always better after they've been here."

Puppies and kittens are naturally affectionate, and having something warm and soft to cuddle is soothing to many people with Alzheimer's. A pet is a big responsibility, however, and one that the person with Alzheimer's cannot be expected to share for much time. Ask yourself if you can reasonably handle caring for a pet too.

One alternative to having your own pet is to enroll in a visiting-pet program, usually offered by veterinary associations or animal shelters. Or if you know people who work all day and leave their pets at home, perhaps they would be willing to drop off a dog or cat in the morning and pick it up after work. If you plan to bring your own or someone else's pet into your home, consult a veterinarian to find out which breeds tend to have good dispositions.

RECREATIONAL ACTIVITIES AND HOBBIES

During the early stages of the disease, those who have always enjoyed participating in particular games, arts and crafts, or hobbies can usually continue to participate with little difficulty, especially if the activity is one they learned many years ago. Ted's wife, Naomi, learned mah-jongg when she was in her twenties and has played regularly for more than forty years. "She can't drive anymore because she gets lost or forgets where she's going," says Ted, "but she still plays a mean game of mahjongg!"

General Tips for Helping with Recreational Activities

As manual dexterity and memory diminish, individuals with Alzheimer's may become angry or frustrated at their inability to perform tasks they could do easily before the disease. "Jennifer loves to make jigsaw puzzles," says Donald. "Those with fifteen hundred pieces used to be her favorite. Now she does much easier ones, with one hundred or fifty pieces. I don't know how she'll react to children's puzzles that have only ten or twelve pieces when she reaches that stage."

Hobbies that require tools, toxic substances, or machinery, such as woodworking, sewing, knitting, painting, or model building, will eventually be too dangerous for the person to pursue. You can help create alternatives by trying some of the following strategies:

- Make the activity less complicated, as Donald did.
- Replace a painter's toxic paints with watercolors, or a model maker's glue with nontoxic pastes.
- People who have enjoyed sewing or knitting could be encouraged to make rag dolls, sock animals, yarn ornaments, or other items that don't require sewing. For example Holly found a local charity that makes and distributes homemade stuffed toys for children with disabilities. She told the volunteer coordinator that her mother, Josephine, could stuff the toys and tie on the bows. Holly takes Josephine to the center twice a week for two to three hours to work on the toys.

- Sculptors and potters can use modeling clay and a blunt plastic tool to continue their hobbies.
- Gardeners should be given plastic tools to use rather than sharp metal ones. If a large plot is too much for them to handle, have them work in window boxes, or place several large planters on the porch.
- People who like to read will not be able to concentrate on novels or long articles. Suggest short stories, poetry, or young-adult fiction. Most libraries carry large-print books, which are helpful for people with vision problems. Also consider short stories on tape.
- People who enjoy collecting such items as antiques, old bottles, stamps, and coins may not be able to actively acquire these items, but they can look at books and magazines about their collectibles. Many of these books are available in local libraries.
- Rent videos or borrow them free from the library for movie buffs who are unable to go to movie theaters.
- Armchair traveling can replace the real thing. Many excellent travelogue videos can be borrowed from a library or travel agency.
- Of course not everyone will be happy doing a scaled-down version of his or her hobby. Some will feel resentment or anger if you suggest they make a change. "Jeremy is furious that he can't do his woodworking the way he used to," said Gail. "But all those tools are too dangerous. I suggested he assemble precut kits that use glue, but he refused. I know it's not the same. He used to make such beautiful things."

Patience and understanding are needed under these circumstances. Reassure the person that you understand his or her frustration. Encourage him or her not to dwell on tasks that can no longer be performed.

Miscellaneous Activities

The following activities are enjoyable for many people with Alzheimer's. Some may argue that these suggestions are "busywork" or too infantile for adults. For individuals who are still able to recognize such items or activities as childish (dolls, plastic cars and trucks, coloring books), this is true. However, for those in the later stages of disease, functioning and comprehension are increasingly limited, and very simple activities may give them pleasure.

Use your judgment regarding the person's mental and emotional state when suggesting these activities. Also pay attention to preferences. If someone is unwilling to engage in a particular activity, don't insist.

- *Beanbag toss.* The target for this activity can be as simple as a white line on the floor. This is something young children can enjoy with a grandparent.
- *Collages.* Collect a variety of materials for the person to cut (using child's scissors) and paste: colorful pictures from old magazines, the fronts of used greeting cards, fabric scraps, buttons, construction paper.
- *Dried flowers and leaves.* Collect and press flowers and leaves. These can be pasted into scrapbooks or onto boards.
- *Folding fabrics.* Gather pieces of different textures—velvet, silk, wool, corduroy, leather, plush, taffeta, and so on. Handling and stroking fabric can be soothing.
- *Bird-watching.* "We hung two bird feeders on the

back porch," said Gabe. "My mother enjoys filling the feeders every morning and sitting and watching the birds fly in to eat. She sits there for several hours, quite content."

- *Drawing and painting.* Provide nontoxic paints or crayons and large sheets of butcher paper.
- *Coloring.* Coloring books and crayons can keep the person occupied for hours. This is another good activity for young children to share with their grandparent.

Remember, helping the person with Alzheimer's stay as active and alert as possible will make you both feel better, and may even slow the course of the disease somewhat. Eventually, however, respite care and other living arrangements may need to be considered. These issues are covered in the next chapter.

NINE

When to Consider Other Living Arrangements

Colette came into the support group meeting after everyone else was seated. Several women made room for her and held her hand after she sat down. She smiled uncertainly and said, "Today I put Andy into a nursing home. I feel terrible and relieved at the same time. After being together for forty-four years, he doesn't even know who I am. I can't take care of him anymore."

Nearly every caregiver gets to a point where he or she needs to find either part-time or permanent full-time outside care for the person with Alzheimer's. Many are like Colette, whose own less-than-perfect health doesn't allow her to care for her husband any longer. Working children who care for an ailing parent also need to utilize outside care.

Eventually most caregivers must find a permanent alternative to home care. Making this decision is never easy, and you're likely to have very mixed feelings during the process. In this chapter we'll explore the decision-making process and suggest strategies for selecting temporary, part-time, and permanent alternatives to full-time home care.

DECIDING TO GET HELP

Deciding to seek additional help and ultimately to place the person you're caring for in a nursing home or other long-term facility can be a difficult, stressful process. Often it comes after you have provided years of home care and undergone emotional strain, personal sacrifice, and financial burden, buoyed by the fact that despite the hardships, you were at least caring for the person yourself, in the home environment.

Before considering long-term-care outside the home, you may decide to see what assistance is available to enable the person to remain at home, at least partially in your care. Accepting that you can no longer do everything necessary to provide the person with Alzheimer's with optimal care yourself is difficult enough, because accepting the fact that the person needs more help also means accepting that the disease is progressing and is taking more of a toll than before. This can be a difficult reality to face—but a necessary one. It is better to own up to the fact that you need additional help than to risk harming your own health by attempting to exceed your limitations, or venting your frustrations on the person you're caring for. Choices such as having someone come into your home, taking advantage of adult day care, or making use of short-stay residential care can be options at this point.

There comes a time, however, when the person will need the intensive, round-the-clock care provided by a nursing home or other long-term-care facility. And no matter how obvious the need, you may feel uncertain and guilty about taking this step. Are you making the right choice? Is there anything else you can do or could have done?

It is important to accept and deal with your feelings of ambivalence and guilt. Although the decision is painful, there must be the realization that you have done the best you could and that now the person needs a higher professional level of care than you can provide.

It is also vital to realize that placing the care of the person with Alzheimer's in the hands of professionals does not mean that you have no further responsibilities with respect to the person's care and well-being. In fact your presence and ability to express affection—whether care continues in the home or you use day care or a long-term facility—will help the person with Alzheimer's feel secure, wanted, and important to others.

HAVING SOMEONE COME INTO YOUR HOME

Various types of home-care workers can assist you in caring for the person with Alzheimer's so that he or she can remain at home as long as possible, if that is what you desire. A homemaker can assist with tasks such as cooking, laundry, and cleaning; a home health worker can help the person bathe, dress, eat, and take care of personal hygiene. A paid companion can supervise the person and may help engage him or her in therapeutic or recreational activities. To find such workers, get referrals from your local Alzheimer's Association chapter, Office of Aging, or members of your support group.

Nurses and other professionals such as a physical therapist or social worker may also be sent to the home by visiting-nurse and home-health agencies. It is important to realize, however, that the services of these workers (as well as homemakers and companions) may not be covered by insurance (for example, Medicare and Medicaid will pay for home nursing care only under strictly defined circumstances). Therefore you must understand all costs associated with hiring such workers and determine in advance whether you can afford them (see chapter 10 for advice on financial planning).

If you decide to hire someone privately rather than from an agency, be aware that you are legally responsible for acting as an employer. You should check the person's licenses and references, follow state and federal payroll requirements (including payment of Social Security), and file the appropriate government forms. Again, be sure to check with your insurance company regarding coverage for the services of these workers.

Your success with a home-care worker depends on your knowing exactly what you need and expect from the person and conveying those expectations clearly from the outset. Before hiring anyone, ask yourself the following questions:

- What specific duties do I need this person to perform?
- How many hours per day and days per week do I need this individual?
- Do I need live-in help?
- Will insurance cover the cost? If not, how will I pay for this type of assistance?

Here are some additional points to remember when bringing a professional helper into your home:

- Make sure both you and the home-care worker have a clear understanding of the chores to be done. Make a list of the agreed-upon tasks and post it in the kitchen or other area of your home.
- If the person you're caring for needs to take medication, and administering it is one of the home-care worker's responsibilities, be sure to post the medication schedule to avoid confusion.
- If the home-care worker is responsible for bathing the person with Alzheimer's, make sure he or she does so gently and thoroughly.
- Keep a record of the hours worked and check them against the agency's or worker's bills.

ADULT-DAY-CARE FACILITIES

Adult-day-care facilities are either publicly or privately run centers that offer recreational activities, an opportunity for people with Alzheimer's to socialize and make new friends, and an environment where they may feel less pressure to perform and thus can feel better about themselves. "The day-care center has been a lifesaver for me," said Drew. "Elizabeth seems to be well cared for, she's with other people like herself, and there are so many activities for her to participate in. They know how to handle her when she gets agitated. I don't have the strength to take care of her full-time, and I know that eventually I'll have to make permanent arrangements for her when she can't go to the center anymore."

Be aware that the services in these centers can vary greatly. Some offer nursing and counseling services as well as therapeutic and recreational activities. Days and hours of operation vary. In some centers transportation and hot meals are provided; others offer neither of these amenities. Also, some day-care centers do not take people with severe behavior problems, or those who are incontinent or need other specialized medical care.

Shop carefully for an adult-day-care center that suits your needs. Consider the following factors:

- *Hours of operation.* Some centers are open seven days a week; others only five or less. While some open as early as six A.M. and stay open until evening, others follow a nine-to-five schedule.
- *Staffing.* Make an appointment with the administrator or supervisor and arrange a formal visit. Ask what the staff-participant ratio is and how many staff members are specifically trained to deal with people with Alzheimer's. Meet the staff and observe how they interact with the participants.
- *Level of care.* As noted earlier, some centers accept individuals who are incontinent; others will not. Some have separate programs for people with Alzheimer's while others bring together people with other dementias and stroke. Not all centers can handle people who wander or who are agitated. Others will not take persons who cannot walk independently. Ask the administrator or supervisor for a list of behaviors they will and will not accept.
- *Activities.* Melanie's father loves to sing, so it was important that the day-care center she chose have a sing-along or choral group. Drew's wife, Elizabeth, used to sew all her own clothes, so Drew found a center with a program in which members make rag dolls for an area children's shelter. Individuals who are mildly impaired

may want to take advantage of shopping or movie excursions offered by some day-care centers.

- *Appearance.* Are the grounds pleasant? Can participants go outside in a supervised, secured area? Visit the center during different times of day. Check the bathrooms and lunch areas for cleanliness. Ask to see their menus and tour the kitchen.

- *Cost.* Centers run by the city, county, state, or a university often charge nominal fees, or may even be free of charge. Some may charge a minimal fee for lunch and snacks. Fees for private centers vary widely. However, it is important to recognize that higher cost does not necessarily translate into better care. Many low-cost centers are funded by endowments and grants and provide quality care.

- *Caregiver's concerns.* Are you permitted to stay with the person and participate in the activities? Until her father was accustomed to the center, Jill knew he would be upset if she just dropped him off every morning on her way to work. "I asked the center's supervisors if I could stay with him for an hour or two for the first few days. They said they encouraged it, so I requested a few mornings off at work. I'm so glad I did. Dad's adjusted well, and he's not anxious when I leave. I also had a chance to meet other caregivers."

- *Convenience.* Is the center located near your home or place of business? Is transportation provided?

To find adult-day-care centers, ask for recommendations from your physician, nurse, social worker, your local Alzheimer's Association chapter, or people in your support group. Look in the Yellow Pages under "Day Care—Adult," "Senior-Citizen Services," or "Nursing

Homes" and in the Resource Guide (chapter 12). For additional information, contact the National Institution on Adult Day Care, 600 Maryland Avenue S.W., Washington, D.C. 20024.

FOSTER CARE

Elderly foster care enables some people with Alzheimer's to be cared for in a foster home, where they receive supervision, a room, meals, and transportation to medical facilities. Foster families are paid by the state, and it is important to select a family that maintains an attitude of respect and caring for those in their charge. Sometimes you may negotiate on your own with a foster home to take the person with Alzheimer's on a short-term basis, to enable you to take some time for yourself for a weekend, a week, or a few weeks.

LIFE-CARE FACILITIES

For an initial down payment plus a monthly charge and, at times, added service fees for nursing, life-care facilities provide a living situation similar to that of a retirement community. Residents receive care for the remainder of their lives, and as their health declines, they are moved to skilled nursing settings within the facility. Generally this is an option for people who have considerable assets.

Not every life-care facility offers the same level of nursing care, however, and some may not provide care for people with Alzheimer's. Check carefully before committing to such an arrangement. Examine the contract and policies carefully. Contact your state consumer-protection office or attorney general's office regarding the laws covering life-care fees in your state. You may want to have an attorney experienced in elder law review any papers before you sign them (see the next chapter for more advice on legal issues).

NURSING HOMES

A nursing home, also known as a skilled-care facility, is an alternative for people who need continuous medical and nursing care including vital-sign monitoring, supervision, administration of medicines, and assistance with daily-living activities. The facility provides nursing care around the clock, with a physician on staff or on call.

Theodore met with a social worker two days after his wife was diagnosed with Alzheimer's. "She said one thing we needed to talk about was finding a nursing home. 'But Ursula won't need a nursing home for years,' I said. Then she told me that's probably how long it would take to find a good one. That comment astounded me. But I got moving right away."

Ideally you should begin the process of choosing a nursing home or other alternative living arrangement immediately after the diagnosis of probable Alzheimer's disease is made. If that sounds too soon, consider that most nursing homes have a waiting list and that not all homes have Alzheimer units. Choosing a facility is time-consuming, and it is best to survey alternatives before you feel pressured into making a hasty decision and settling for a home you really don't care for.

Types of Nursing Homes

Nursing homes fall into one of three basic categories: private for-profit facilities; voluntary homes operated by a religious or communal organization; and nonprofit public homes run by government agencies. All nursing homes must meet state and local standards, and each state has its own quality-assurance system.

Cost

Most people end up paying for nursing-home care out of their own pockets unless they are impoverished, in which case Medicaid may cover many of the costs. Insurance policies typically have clauses that exclude care for diseases such as Alzheimer's, although some will cover limited nursing-home care. Medicare is not designed to cover long-term care in a nursing home, but it does offer partial coverage for a limited time in certain cases where an individual has a coexisting condition (for example, diabetes, heart failure) that requires nursing care. The nursing home must be Medicare-certified in order for your claim to be considered. Medicaid is designed to cover long-term custodial care, but its eligibility criteria are strict. Because the requirements and policies for these programs change frequently, it is strongly recommended that you consult an attorney who is familiar with Medicare and Medicaid. Contact your local Alzheimer's Association for more information.

The Selection Process

Referrals to nursing homes can come from your physician, social workers, local Alzheimer's Association office, and perhaps most helpful of all, other caregivers who have a family member or spouse in a nursing facility. Once you have a few homes on your list, contact the administrator at each one and find out about costs and financial arrangements, how many beds are available, the level of care available, and the length of the waiting list.

Set up an appointment with the administrator to tour each facility at least once, preferably two or three times if you are seriously considering it. Make the second and third visits unannounced and at different times of the day —during meals and activity times. Bring a relative, another caregiver, or a member of the Alzheimer's Association with you to help.

Doreen brought along a woman from her Alzheimer's support group when she visited the first nursing home. "I felt overwhelmed when I first walked in," she said. "It was a good thing I had Ruth with me. The administrators were very accommodating, and they helped me relax. They showed us the activity rooms, residents' rooms, and dining halls. The residents looked well groomed. Ruth asked to see the residents' bathrooms. I didn't think to ask that! We liked what we saw that day, but we need to go back. The administrator said we were welcome anytime."

Questions to Ask

In addition to observing the facility, it is important to sit down with the administrator and, if possible, with various staff members, to discuss your concerns. To get the most out of your discussions, bring a list of questions with you. Remember, several heads are better than one. Discuss your questions and concerns with family, other caregivers, social workers, your physician, and clergy. If the person with Alzheimer's is in the early stages of disease and is willing, he or she can also help with the decision. Any one of these individuals may raise questions or make observations you may miss.

- *Fees:* Is the nursing home certified to accept Medicare or Medicaid? Will they continue to care for a person who switches from private pay to Medicaid? What services are included in the basic fee and which are extra? (Ask for a copy of the financial arrangements; some homes charge additional fees for physical therapy, incontinence pads, medications, laundry services, hairdresser, and other services.) Are refunds available for unused services?
- *Medical care:* What kind of medical care does the facility provide? Is there a special Alzheimer's unit? What is their policy with respect to physical restraints and sedation? (Ask to see their written policy on use of restraints and psychoactive drugs.) How often do residents receive checkups? How are wanderers handled? How is incontinence handled? Are dental care and eye care offered? Can you help prepare the resident's care plan? Which hospital would the resident be taken to in case of emergency?
- *Staff:* How many staff are specially trained to handle Alzheimer's patients? How many physicians and skilled nurses are on staff? How much experience do social workers and recreational staff have with Alzheimer's res-

idents? How many residents must each aide care for? Do the staff members seem friendly? Harried? How do they interact with the residents?

Doreen had visited three nursing homes and was considering two of them. On her second visit to Home A she paid particular attention to the staff. "Many of them didn't look too happy," she said. "A few of them didn't address the residents by name and seemed annoyed when they walked too slowly. I hadn't noticed these things the first time I was there. I asked a few aides how long they had worked there, and all three said less than a year. 'This place has a revolving door,' one of them told me. I asked a friend who works at an area hospital if she knew what the turnover was like there, and she confirmed that it was high."

- *Environment:* What is the overall atmosphere when you walk into the nursing home—dismal, cheerful, unusually quiet? Are the hallways and rooms bright and cheerful? Are the dining halls and kitchen areas clean? Are the residents' bathrooms clean and equipped with grab bars and handrails? Are the halls and rooms safe (nonskid flooring) for walkers and wheelchairs? Are the beds comfortable?
- *Regulations:* Does the facility have a current state license? Does the administrator have a current license from the state? (If the answer to either of these questions is no, do not consider the facility.) All the proper licenses issued by the state (fire safety, type of staff, sufficient number of staff to attend to residents, proper nutrition) should be displayed; if not, ask to see them and inquire about any recent failed inspections and the reason for each. Is the facility accredited by the Joint Commission on Accreditation of Hospitals or the American Health

Care Association? These two review organizations ensure quality care in nursing facilities.

- *Residents:* Do the residents seem happy? Can residents wear their own clothes? Are many of them restrained? Do they seem overly sedated? Are their clothes clean? Are they well groomed?

What types of activities are planned? Do residents get enough exercise? Are there supervised, secure outdoor areas? Do residents have access to television, radio, a library, movies? Are religious services offered? Can caregivers join residents in their activities?

- *Food:* Is the food appetizing and nutritious? Are special diets offered? Are Alzheimer's residents fed by hand when they can no longer feed themselves? What is the facility's policy on tube feeding?

Will they accommodate special requests? "My wife must have grapefruit every morning or she gets extremely upset," said Abe. "This has been going on for more than two years. When I told the administrator that, he said, 'Sometimes we can break people of these little habits.' For my wife it's not a little habit, and he'd see how big a deal it is if he didn't give her grapefruit. I guess you can say I didn't choose that place because of grapefruit."

- *Visitors:* Are visiting hours liberal or restricted to narrow times? Is there enough space for privacy during visits? Are children allowed to visit? Is it convenient (distance, parking) for you to visit?

- *Residents' rights:* Does the facility have a residents' council where you can voice your concerns and complaints and be assured they will reach the administration? Is there a family council? Can you meet with the social worker regularly to discuss the resident and his or her care? How is the patient's bill of rights carried out in the facility? (These rights are federally mandated; you are entitled to receive a copy.)

• *Policy on terminal care:* What is the facility's policy regarding life-sustaining measures? (Laws differ by state, so you will want to check what your state requires of nursing homes.) Can you be assured that the resident's advance directives are part of his or her medical chart?

Before You Sign

Making a final decision on a nursing home is a particularly stressful time for you, so be sure to take your time before making a commitment. Before you sign the contract, make sure you understand everything it says. If possible, have an attorney review the agreement. The contract should clearly spell out the following:

• The nature of medical care to be provided to the potential resident (care by physicians, nurses, therapists; prescriptions; any required therapy).
• What the monthly rate covers (i.e., meals, lodging, laundry, nursing services, recreational programs, nonprescription medical supplies) and what items or services are extra (i.e., personal items, television).
• Reasons for transfer or discharge, and notification procedure should transfer become necessary.

STATE MENTAL HOSPITALS

Occasionally individuals with Alzheimer's have severe behavior problems that make it impossible for them to be placed in a nursing home, or they may have to be transferred after placement.

"My brother, Jules, became combative after three months in the nursing home," said Lowell. "He attacked several patients, and the staff had to restrain him physically. Now they want me to make other arrangements. Will he have to go to the state mental hospital? I've heard nothing but horror stories about those places."

Not all state mental hospitals deserve a "snake pit" reputation. Some have good programs for treating severe behavior problems that make the person a danger to others or to himself or herself; others do provide a poorer quality of care than nursing homes or other facilities. In any case, since the federal government has mandated that state hospitals reduce their geriatric patient load, the hospital in your state may not be in a position to accept a new patient. Signatures of a psychiatrist and a physician are required to have a person admitted to a state mental hospital, but even then you may not be able to get a bed for the person.

The financial burden for individuals who are admitted to the state mental hospital is on the family, though costs are generally considerably less than for a nursing home. Consult with your social worker, congressional representative, and Alzheimer's Association representative for assistance.

If the person is displaying problem behaviors, there are other avenues you can try before contemplating placement in a state hospital. Some states have programs that bring together psychiatrists, social workers, and nurses who evaluate individuals with severe behavior problems, prescribe medications, and train the nursing-home staff to deal with the person. A representative of the

Alzheimer's Association or your social worker will know if your state has such a program. Lowell's state did not have this program. However, the Alzheimer's Association representative suggested he contact his congressional representative and his social worker so that together they could put together a team that would accomplish the same goal. Lowell informed the nursing home of his efforts. Within a few weeks Jules had been evaluated by a psychiatrist, who prescribed appropriate sedatives, and two staff members received specialized patient-care training. As a result Jules was allowed to remain at the nursing home.

HOSPICES

Individuals who are in the terminal stage of Alzheimer's and have a prognosis of six months or less may be placed in a hospice. A hospice offers a caring environment where people with Alzheimer's are kept comfortable and permitted to die with dignity, and a place where caregivers and their families can receive support and counseling.

Some aspects of hospice care may be available at home through visiting nurses and other services, so that the individual may be permitted to spend his or her final months in a familiar and loving setting.

TEN

Financial and Legal Concerns

"Two weeks after Horace was diagnosed with Alzheimer's, we talked to a social worker our physician had recommended. She told us we were very smart to think ahead and that we were fortunate Horace could still make his own financial and legal decisions. That was three years ago, and back then I didn't feel very fortunate. Today I realize she was right. We found a lawyer to help us sort out our finances and insurance and plan for our future. Today Horace no longer knows who I am. He's in a nursing home, and I live in a little apartment nearby so that I can visit him every day. It hurts. But at least I know his wishes are being respected."

—*Carole*

Although tackling financial and legal matters may be the last thing you want to do after hearing the diagnosis of Alzheimer's disease, it is an essential step. It is important to plan now for the future care of the person with Alzheimer's. If the individual is mentally capable of sharing this responsibility, so much the better. Early attention to these issues can prevent problems later in the course of the disease, when the person is no longer mentally competent. Prompt action will also let you know the person's wishes are being respected and will relieve you of the burden of second-guessing later in the disease process.

Presenting a complete description of the many complex issues involved in these areas is beyond the scope of this book; moreover laws regarding competency and incompetency vary from state to state. However, in this chapter we will provide an overview of areas of key concern, a look at your options, and explanations of special financial and legal terminology. We'll also tell you how to select professionals to help with your particular needs and requirements.

FINDING PROFESSIONAL HELP

Financial and legal professionals can help you manage the assets of the person with Alzheimer's and help you make long-range financial plans. When selecting an attorney, financial planner, accountant, or other professional, be sure he or she is familiar with elder law, trusts, estate law, Medicare and Medicaid provisions, and long-term-care financing.

You can find and select these professionals in much the same way as you would select a physician or other health care provider (see chapter 6). Ask other caregivers or support-group members for references. Also contact your local Alzheimer's Association chapter, Office of Aging, or organizations listed in the Resource Guide (chapter 12) of this book. Free or low-cost financial and legal services are available in most states.

When calling for an appointment, assess whether the attitude of the professional's staff is cordial, helpful, and concerned. This can provide clues about how your concerns will be handled. Also ask about fees (including whether you are charged for phone consultations) and hours.

Ask what information and material you should bring with you to the meeting. This may include details about the income, bank accounts, loans, investments, insurance policies, mortgages, trusts, pensions, and will of the person with Alzheimer's. You may need to bring the person's birth certificate and, if appropriate, papers to confirm that the person is widowed or divorced. A list of the spouse's assets is also required in most cases.

Make a list of questions to ask during the meeting. Take notes or tape responses to your questions.

If the person with Alzheimer's is mentally competent, he or she should go with you. You may want to bring along a family member or friend to assist you during this stressful time.

LEGAL MATTERS

Eventually people with Alzheimer's lose the ability to make decisions concerning their own medical, legal, and financial status. Various types of legal documents may be prepared to protect them and permit them to legally designate a person of their choice to handle their affairs for them. These documents include a will, durable power of attorney, guardianship, living trust, living will, and health care proxy.

Will

If the person with Alzheimer's is mentally competent but has not prepared a will as yet, one should be prepared as soon as possible. For a will to be valid, the person making it (the testator) must be able to:

- Understand the nature and extent of the property being bequeathed
- Present a reasonable plan for how the property should be distributed
- Understand the relationship between himself or herself and the people who will receive the property
- And keep all these factors in mind at the time the will is executed

People with Alzheimer's often go in and out of lucid periods. A good time to prepare a will is during a lucid period. "Nicholas had his good and bad days," said his wife, Nettie. "To assure the validity of his will, we had a psychiatrist examine him at the time the will was executed to attest to his competency."

Your lawyer may recommend such precautionary measures if you believe the will may be contested by potential heirs.

Power of Attorney

A regular power of attorney (one that is not durable) gives a designated person the authority to act on the patient's behalf at any time before the patient becomes incapacitated, but not afterward. The preferred power of attorney for someone with Alzheimer's is a durable power of attorney, since the disease is progressive, and the person may become incapacitated at any time.

Springing/Durable Power of Attorney

Unlike a regular power of attorney, which becomes void when the signer becomes mentally incapacitated, a springing or durable power of attorney gives the designated person (known as *the agent* or *attorney in fact*) the power to act and sign documents on behalf of the person with Alzheimer's (known as *the principal*) after he or she is declared mentally incompetent. In the case of Douglas and Miriam, Douglas signed a durable power of attorney that named his wife "attorney in fact." He continued to be involved in their financial and legal decisions for several years until he was no longer competent; then Miriam took over. Durable power of attorney may be assigned to any person of legal age—a spouse, sibling, child, or other adult.

Guardianship

When a person with Alzheimer's is mentally incompetent or unwilling to assign a power of attorney, you must have a lawyer petition the court for a guardianship of property (also called a *conservatorship*). After a court hearing, the judge decides whether the person is mentally capable of handling his or her own property and financial affairs. If not, a guardian or conservator is assigned to care for the property under supervision of the court. If you are named a conservator, you must file periodic reports to the court on the person's financial status.

Another type of guardianship is guardianship of the person. A person may require medical or nursing-home care and be unable or unwilling to make the decisions necessary to secure that care. Generally a spouse or next of kin can make such decisions without the court assigning a guardian. Occasionally, however, if there is a dispute among family members about the individual's care, some states will request a guardianship of the person or give a court order that the care be provided.

Living Trust

A living trust allows individuals (called *grantors*) to preserve their resources during and after their lifetime. The grantor names one or more persons, a bank, or both, as trustee(s).

"My father had a lot of assets, and the lawyer suggested he set up a living trust," said Colleen. "Dad got to specify how he wanted his money spent during the remainder of his lifetime. This was important to him, and I was glad that his wishes were respected."

By law, the trustee(s) must adhere to the guidelines spelled out in the trust by the grantor regarding the way in which assets are to be managed. Assets can be dispensed throughout the person's lifetime, or part or all can be preserved for after the person's death.

Living Will

A living will allows an individual to clearly state his or her wishes regarding the use of life-sustaining treatment and how health care decisions should be made in the event of mental incapacity. "Craig and I had often discussed getting a living will, but we didn't do anything about it until he was diagnosed with Alzheimer's," said Anne. "We both have very strong feelings about not wanting needles and tubes to be the only things keeping us alive."

Most, but not all, states recognize living wills. Discuss your options with your lawyer.

Health Care Proxy

A health care proxy allows an individual to authorize a spouse, adult child, or other adult to make health care decisions for him or her in the event the person becomes mentally incompetent. It can be used to make decisions about any health care measure, not just life-sustaining treatment.

Medicaid regulations prohibit family members from making treatment decisions for people who are mentally incapacitated unless a court guardian has been assigned or the patient has signed a health care proxy. Thus having a proxy can prevent expensive court proceedings and delays in medical treatment in the future. Remember, however, that a health care proxy can govern health decisions only. The person is not designated to make financial decisions unless he or she also has power of attorney or guardianship.

Other Legal Matters

If the person you're caring for inadvertently breaks the law, he or she may still be held responsible for these actions. Geoff explained what happened to his brother. "Jake had wandered off, and the whole family was looking for him. The police found him the next day, wandering in the park, confused, with his pants down around his ankles. Fortunately the police knew about his condition and he wasn't arrested."

Occasionally people with Alzheimer's may have a "run-in" with the law. Wandering and exposing themselves are two common situations when this may occur. Generally people must show criminal intent when committing an act that is considered a crime, and this then falls under the auspices of criminal law. When a person has Alzheimer's disease, his or her legal responsibility is lessened. This will not prevent the police from arresting or holding an individual if an apparent crime has been committed, however. Nor does it release you from your responsibility to try to prevent such incidents.

Civil matters have their own rules. "Joseph took the car keys and drove the car into the side of the neighbor's house," said his wife. "No one was hurt, but we have to pay for the damages." Regardless of their mental condition, people with Alzheimer's, as well as their family, may be liable for damages.

Soon after the diagnosis of Alzheimer's is made, you may want to review your insurance policies to be certain they cover damages that may be attributed directly to the disease. Your insurance agent can help you with your questions.

Another legal matter to consider is ownership of the property of the person with Alzheimer's. It might be preferable to transfer title of all properties, including jointly owned properties, to a spouse, family member, or friend. However, transferring assets is a step that should be taken only after consideration of tax and other important implications.

Estate Planning

As the disease progresses and the patient becomes more dependent upon you, the caregiver, you may be concerned about the patient's well-being or protection in the event you can no longer provide care. Professional assistance from a lawyer and financial specialist should enable you to plan an arrangement that will meet both your needs.

FINANCIAL ASSESSMENT

Before you and the person with Alzheimer's can begin to plan for the future, you need to have a good understanding of his or her current financial status and the costs of current and future care. "The social worker said we needed to start thinking about in-home care and nursing-home care for my mother," said Georgia. "We didn't know where to begin. We knew the cost of nursing-home care was staggering, and I wasn't sure how we could pay for it." If you are a spouse of a person with Alzheimer's, you must also plan for your own financial future.

Determining Current Financial Status

To determine the person's current financial condition, take the following steps:

- Add all earned and unearned income: salary, pensions, Social Security, interest and dividends, and rental income.
- List current liabilities: monthly living expenses (rent

or mortgage, taxes, utilities, food, transportation, medications, subscriptions, recreation, etc.), credit card balances, insurance and taxes, all outstanding debts.

• Subtract total liabilities from total income for the net monthly income figure (the amount of money available after all expenses are paid).

• Tally all assets, which may include stocks and bonds, real estate, bank and credit union accounts, health and life insurance, and certificates of deposit. This figure, in addition to net income, is the one you will need when applying for most financial-assistance programs. If you are the spouse of the person with Alzheimer's, your assets and income may count as well, depending on the program.

Calculating Costs of Care

The anticipated costs of care of the person with Alzheimer's—both at home and in a long-term facility—should be calculated as soon as possible. Because disease progression varies and people may require care for many years, these costs can be unpredictable and substantial. Some individuals stay at home for several years, while others require nursing-home care within a year or two of diagnosis. Consider the following factors when making your calculations:

• *Income:* Will income be lost because the person with Alzheimer's has to leave his or her job? Will he or she retain retirement or disability benefits? Will you need to leave your job in order to care for the person?

• *Housing:* What living arrangements will need to be made: life-care facility, halfway house, moving in with you? If the person can stay in his or her own home, will modifications need to be made (ramps for a wheelchair, new locks, handrails, safety features in the bathroom and kitchen)? Will you and the person you're caring for need to move to a home that is safer and more convenient (closer to services, needing less maintenance)?

• *Medical:* Will you need any of the following: home nurses, prescriptions, physicians' visits, psychiatric evaluations, counseling, medical supplies and devices (wheelchair, shower chair, hospital bed, incontinence products), physical or occupational therapy? Will your insurance cover any of these needs? If not, how will you pay for these items and services?

• *Home help and respite care:* Will you need the services of a home health care worker or housekeeper? Will you take the person with Alzheimer's to adult day care or a respite program?

• *Food and transportation:* Will you need help preparing meals, or will you have meals brought in? Are you able to drive? Is alternative transportation available, and how much will it cost?

• *Legal and financial costs:* Will you need help preparing your taxes? Will you have to prepare taxes for the person you're caring for? Will you need to hire a lawyer and/or financial adviser?

• *Nursing-home costs:* Do you know the average cost of nursing-home care in your area? Do you know the services and items for which you will be charged extra?

How to Pay for Medical Care

Three types of medical insurance are available for at-home and nursing-home care of people with Alzheimer's:

Medicare, Medicaid, and private health and major-medical insurance. Since regulations vary from state to state and health care reform is likely to affect these options, check with an Alzheimer's Association representative, a lawyer who specializes in elder law, or your local Office of Aging for the latest information on eligibility requirements and reimbursement.

The following overview will help you become familiar with some of the regulations and policies that govern these types of insurance at the time of this writing:

Medicare

To be eligible for Medicare, a person must be sixty-five years or older and eligible for Social Security or Railroad Retirement benefits, or be a disabled person of any age. Medicare covers acute rather than chronic or long-term care. If a person with Alzheimer's becomes acutely and seriously ill and needs nursing care, however, Medicare may cover the acute illness. Maximum coverage is 150 days, and the individual will be required to pay part of the bill (known as a *copayment).*

Medicaid

Medicaid is a complex federal program that is run and funded with your federal and state (and in some cases, city) tax dollars. It may provide coverage of nursing-home care, full-time home health care, and adult day care for people with Alzheimer's and other disabling conditions if the person meets the financial-need requirements. It may also cover inpatient and outpatient hospital care; laboratory and radiology services; most prescription and some nonprescription drugs; physical examinations; and dental, eye, and hearing care.

Generally people become eligible for Medicaid after they have depleted their own resources and assets and are below the federal poverty level. A spouse's income and assets are taken into consideration when determining Medicaid eligibility. This does not mean that a spouse must spend all of his or her resources before the person with Alzheimer's is eligible for Medicaid, however. If assets can be transferred to an adult child, for example, then after some time these assets are not included in eligibility calculations.

Three years ago Lindsey's father transferred the majority of his assets to his daughter's name. He has lived with his daughter for most of that time, and now he needs to be placed in a nursing home. Because his monthly income is below the maximum allowed to qualify for Medicaid, he was admitted to the facility as a Medicaid patient.

Individuals or families who want to transfer assets must do so at least thirty months before the person with Alzheimer's applies for Medicaid. This rule applies to all assets, including the person's home, but does not include transfer of the home to the spouse living in the community.

Both federal and state (and sometimes city) laws govern Medicaid; eligibility requirements are different in every state and change frequently. In some states, for example, spouses and adult children are not legally bound to spend their own resources to support family members in nursing homes. Other states, however, have "relative responsibility laws," which require family members to provide financial support for the person. Because of the complexity of these laws it is best to consult a lawyer or other professional who is knowledgeable about Medicaid regulations.

Private Insurance

Health insurance and major-medical insurance policies differ greatly in terms of coverage, the amount of deductible you must pay, waiting periods, duration of benefits, and exclusions for preexisting or chronic conditions. "My husband has a long-term-care insurance policy he took out many years ago," said Carla, "so I thought I wouldn't have trouble paying for his nursing-home care. Then I discovered that the daily amount it covered is based on 1972 prices! We didn't have an inflation rider on the policy."

Once a person has a diagnosis of Alzheimer's, virtually no insurance company will write a new policy for his or her health care.

However, the person's life insurance policy may be a resource. Some insurance companies will add a long-term-care rider to a life insurance policy, which provides a monthly payout equal to a fixed percentage of the death benefit.

"The insurance agent explained that the long-term-care rider on my father's $100,000 life insurance policy would pay up to 1.5 percent, or $1,500, of the monthly nursing-home costs," said Colleen. "That's only half of the monthly charge, but at least we're halfway there."

Long-term-care riders must be purchased before a person becomes incapacitated. Contact your insurance agent about the current policies of the person with Alzheimer's and how to make the most of them.

Obtaining Financial Assistance

Various federal, state, and private programs are available to assist people with Alzheimer's and their families when they are in financial need. Each program has its own eligibility requirements and restrictions. Unless otherwise noted, more information on these programs may be obtained by contacting your local Department of Welfare, Social Services, or Human Resources.

- *Social Security:* Monthly benefits are paid to retired, disabled, and blind individuals who contributed to the program while they were working. Occasionally payments may also be made to the person's nonworking spouse, widows and widowers, divorcees, dependent parents, and dependent children. Call 1-800-234-5772 for more information.
- *Supplemental Security Income:* This federal program pays a minimum monthly income to individuals who are in financial need and are sixty-five years or older, disabled, or blind. Call 1-800-234-5772.
- *Senior Citizen Rent Increase Exemption:* This program exempts eligible older renters from paying rent increases.
- *Food stamps:* Food stamps can be used in stores and toward meals served at senior centers or delivered to the home.
- *Meals:* Under the Federal Older American Act, programs such as Eating Together Congregate Meals and Home-Delivered Meals are available to individuals fifty-nine years and older regardless of income level. "I go to an Eating Together lunch nearly every day," said Lilly. "They hold it at the church on the corner. The food is good, it's inexpensive, and I've made friends there."

The Meals on Wheels program will send a volunteer to your home with one hot meal per day. There is a nominal charge, which varies depending on location.

- *Home Energy Assistance Program:* Basic or emergency expenses for utilities are paid through this program for people who meet the income requirements.
- *Real Estate Tax Exemption:* Some homeowners may qualify for a reduction in the real estate taxes they pay on their primary residence.
- *Emergency Assistance:* Cash for emergency situations, such as avoiding having the heat in your home turned off because of nonpayment, is provided by this program.
- *Veterans Administration benefits:* These benefits are granted to veterans of the United States Armed Forces, eligible dependents, or survivors of a veteran. Benefits and eligibility are explained in the booklet *Federal Benefits for Veterans and Dependents* (contact the Superintendent of Documents, U.S. Government Printing Office, Washington, D.C. 20402).

Another place to find assistance is your local Department of Aging, which may have programs for elderly people in need of help with home repairs or maintenance, transportation, counseling, and advocacy, among other things. Services are offered at no or low cost for older adults.

In addition the Internal Revenue Service offers various tax breaks or reductions for the elderly, for families who are paying for a parent's medical care, and for some nursing-home care that is not covered by Medicare or Medicaid.

"My mother came to live with us this year," said Doug. "We put in some safety features around the house. My wife also had to quit work to take care of her. Our tax adviser says we can take some deductions for the equipment and for my wife leaving her job. It's going to make a big difference on our return."

Because the laws and requirements governing these situations change yearly, contact the Internal Revenue Service and ask for their latest publications.

ELEVEN

Caring for Yourself

Randall is struggling with many feelings. "I get so angry at Milly that I feel like hitting her. Then I feel like a monster! How could I want to hit her? She's helpless. She's my wife, or what's left of her. That's one reason why I'm angry. I've been robbed. This disease has taken Milly from me, and there's nothing I can do."

"The man I married forty-eight years ago is gone. All that's left is his shell." Laura cared for Fred at home for nearly five years before putting him in a nursing home. "I visit him every day, but he doesn't know it's me. He says, 'Who are you? What do you want?' I used to cry. I don't anymore. I'm numb. I feel like I'm a dead woman visiting a dead man."

The three men and eight women sat in the room around a U-shaped table, drinking coffee and talking among themselves. A tall, well-dressed woman stopped in the doorway but did not enter the room. Instead she stood for a minute and surveyed the group until one of the women called out, "Welcome. I'm Alice. Please join us." The newcomer walked over and shook Alice's outstretched hand. "I'm Julia. I've never been to a support group before, but I don't know where else to turn. Caring for my father is starting to drive me crazy. If I don't talk to someone who understands, I'll explode." Alice held Julia's hand. *"That's why we're here. To talk to one another and to help one another."*

Like you, these people are caregivers—a spouse, son, daughter, sibling, or relative—who is entrusted with the care of a person with Alzheimer's. Every day you face the challenges and frustrations that care entails. You are a bundle of emotions, some of which you might not like or even want to admit you have. Often you are so caught up in caring for the person that you forget you need to take care of yourself too.

This chapter is just for you. In it we look at how to get relief from the emotional and physical stress of caregiving. The demands of caregiving will continue to increase as the disease progresses, and you must be prepared physically and emotionally to meet those demands. You must take care of *you*.

ACCEPTING YOUR FEELINGS

One of the most difficult things for caregivers to do is to accept the fact that they may have so-called negative feelings, such as anger and frustration, as well as committed, caring feelings about the person with Alzheimer's and the caregiver role. Yet you must accept these feelings, and recognize that they are part of a normal reaction to your situation, in order to deal effectively with them.

"I was furious with everyone—the doctor, my husband, myself, God, even the dog. I wanted to blame someone, anyone," said Jill. "I believed no one could possibly understand the way I felt. It hurt to be so angry and helpless and out of control."

Barry looks at his wife, Phyllis, when she's sleeping peacefully and thinks, "I can make it. Things won't get better, but I can make it." Then Phyllis wakes up and babbles on and on for hours. "She doesn't know who I am. I have to shut out her voice by putting on earphones, or I'm afraid I'll scream or hit her. It's horrible to feel this way."

Acceptance—both of your feelings and of your caregiver role—is an ongoing process. One minute you'll feel like you can cope and the next you'll be asking yourself how you'll ever get through the day. Recognize that this pendulum effect is normal.

Penny told her psychologist that she felt as though she were on a merry-go-round. "There are so many feelings swirling around in me," she said. "He told me, 'You have to feel the feelings before you can deal with them.'"

Anger, guilt, embarrassment, and depression are among the most common "negative" feelings experienced by caregivers. Once you accept them, you can deal with them. Let's look at each of these feelings and some specific ideas on how to cope with them.

Anger

Anger is probably the most common emotion experienced by caregivers. Accept that you will feel angry (and frustrated and impatient, which are outgrowths of anger) at various times and to varying degrees. You may end up directing your anger at the survivor, yourself, relatives or friends who may not be supportive, or professionals such as your physician or social worker.

"Sometimes I get so angry at Ron that I find myself shouting at him," said Natalie. "I know he doesn't understand me, but I can't seem to stop myself. Then I feel guilty about screaming at him, which makes me even more upset."

Misdirected anger—lashing out at the person with Alzheimer's or at other people, or chastising yourself—can place great strain on your emotional and physical health. On the other hand, repressed anger—holding down your feelings or numbing yourself—can lead to depression and fatigue and may exacerbate physical ailments, such as stomach disorders and headache. To handle your anger in a healthier way, try the following:

- Remove yourself from the situation, even if only briefly. "Sometimes I just want to scream," say many caregivers. Some of them do go into their rooms and scream into a pillow. Or try what Peggy does: She drives down a country road with the radio blaring while she screams as loudly as she can. The key is to separate yourself from the survivor and go to a safe place—your room, the bathroom, the basement, the garden—and take time for yourself. Punch a pillow, listen to classical music, play the piano, read poetry, take deep breaths.
- Try to avoid situations that you know make you angry. Brittany knows that she nearly explodes when it's time to feed her mother. She enlisted the help of her husband, who feeds his mother-in-law at breakfast, and her twelve-year-old daughter, who helps in the feeding process at dinner.
- Discuss your feelings with someone who is not directly involved with your situation, such as a minister or close friend.

- Incorporate regular exercise into your life, especially some form of vigorous activity that can help you release pent-up anger safely (check with your physician before starting a new exercise program). Natalie bought an aerobic tape that she pops into the VCR whenever she feels the need to let go. Some caregivers take brisk walks or join an exercise class.
- Avoid destructive behaviors. Turning to drugs, alcohol, cigarettes, or food will only make you feel worse in the long run. If you find yourself engaging in such behaviors regularly, you may need professional help.
- If you believe you are angry enough to physically harm the person with Alzheimer's, or if you have already done so, get help *now*. Call an Alzheimer's Association representative or a professional counselor (see the section "Psychotherapy and Counseling" on pages 212–213). Be aware that such abuse is not uncommon among caregivers. Help is out there for you.

Guilt

"Am I doing enough?" "Am I selfish if I want to go out occasionally?" "What if I leave my mother with a friend and something happens while I'm out?" "What will people think if I put my wife in a nursing home?" "Sometimes I wish my husband would die quietly in his sleep; isn't that a horrible thing to wish for?"

Guilt is an emotion that can easily get out of hand. It can cloud your ability to make rational decisions and make you neglect your own health.

Pamela recalls how, many years ago, before her mother was diagnosed with Alzheimer's, "she made me promise I'd never put her into a nursing home. But she's disrupting our entire family. She's verbally abusive to me and the kids. Whenever I think about putting her into a nursing home, I remember my promise, yet I can't live with her anymore."

Caregivers who let guilt adversely affect what they know to be a right decision are hurting themselves as well as the person with Alzheimer's. In Pamela's case her guilt led to such feelings of frustration and anger that she raised her fist one day and nearly hit her mother. Only then did she wake up to the fact that breaking her promise was the wisest thing for all concerned. When she shared her feelings with members of her support group, they reinforced her decision and her responsibility to take care of herself and her family.

The next time you feel guilty, consider the following:

• Did you yell at the person with Alzheimer's or a friend or relative for no justifiable reason? Well, then, accept that you're human. Apologize and realize that next time you can ward off such a reaction, perhaps by using one of the suggestions from the "Anger" section, pages 203–205.

• Did someone say something to you to make you feel as though you're not doing enough, or that your job "isn't very difficult"? Most people who make insensitive remarks don't understand how much energy and time are required of a caregiver. They don't necessarily mean to be cruel.

• Did you go out with friends and feel guilty when you returned home? Why? If you left the individual in capable hands, you have no reason to feel guilty. You must take time to reenergize yourself and unwind.

Depression

Depression is a devastating feeling that can ultimately leave you unable to function.

"For the first few months I was so overwhelmed with talking to the social worker and our attorney and making plans, I didn't think much about myself," said Louisa. "But once I got into an hour-by-hour, day-to-day routine and I realized it was only going to get worse, I began to feel very discouraged and depressed. I had no appetite, and I was tired all the time. A friend suggested I go to a support group, but I wasn't motivated to do anything. I just felt the whole situation was overwhelmingly hopeless."

Fortunately for Louisa, her friend was persistent. After Louisa went to several support-group meetings, she realized she needed to talk with a professional.

"The psychologist helped me find the strength within myself to go on living," said Louisa. "I couldn't cure my husband, but I could at least cure myself. The most I could do for my husband was make him comfortable. The best I could do for myself was to live life to its fullest."

Not everyone needs to seek professional help for depression. Many find adequate relief from talking with other caregivers or family, getting away periodically, hiring in-home assistance, or taking the person with Alzheimer's to an adult-day-care center. If you have tried these measures and are still chronically depressed, professional counseling can help you get back on track.

Embarrassment

The behavior of people with Alzheimer's can be unpredictable and embarrassing. "We were having dinner at a restaurant when my husband got up and stuck his hands into a plate of spaghetti that belonged to a person sitting at the table next to ours. I was humiliated," said Doris.

If you talk with other caregivers in support groups, you will discover that such embarrassing situations are not uncommon. When you and the person with Alzheimer's are with friends, family, or neighbors, explain that the individual has Alzheimer's and may say or do something unusual. Let them know that the individual cannot control his or her behavior. Think of it as a way to educate others about the disease.

PAYING ATTENTION TO YOUR OWN WELL-BEING

The overwhelming responsibility of caring for a person with Alzheimer's often causes caregivers to neglect their own health and well-being. Everyone may see the warning signs—except the caregiver.

"My friend, Rhea, took me aside one day and said, 'I'm worried about you, Loni. You're tired and depressed all the time. You don't talk to anyone. I'm not trying to pry, but I know your mother is a tremendous burden. Is there something I can do?' At first I was angry, but then I realized she was right. I wasn't taking care of myself."

True, every person has his or her own tolerance level and way of responding to stress. Some people can change soiled bedclothes with minimal distress, for example, while others find this task repulsive and must find someone else to do it for them. But no matter how much tolerance you may have, you are not a superperson. Eventually caregiving will take its toll. It is better to recognize the signs of burnout early and take a break than to let stress and exhaustion build up until you can't take it any longer.

Take some time to assess your feelings and behavior honestly. Become aware of how you are reacting to the daily tasks of caregiving. Signals that you need a break include: fatigue; wanting to hit or actually hitting the person with Alzheimer's; weight loss or gain; sleeplessness; feeling overwhelmed most of the time; increased alcohol use; feeling isolated, trapped, or depressed; having temper tantrums, crying spells, difficulty making decisions, and thoughts of suicide.

TAKING ACTION TO RELIEVE STRESS

Once you recognize the need for a break, it is important to take action.

"Rhea was my wakeup call," said Loni. "She made me stop and think. I wasn't taking time to cook for myself because I was worn out trying to get my mother to eat. And she gets up at night, which means I wasn't sleeping. I felt like I wanted to cry most of the time. Once I thought about it, I realized I needed to do something."

That "something" is whatever you must do to cope with the stress and ensure that you regain—and maintain—your emotional and physical health. For Rhea this meant making time to prepare nutritious meals for herself, taking naps on days when she didn't sleep well the night before, and asking her sister to come over to her house once a week to take care of their mother.

In most instances, making just one change in your caregiving role won't be sufficient. For example eating better is a good start, but if you constantly feel guilty about taking your husband to a day-care center while you go to work, or if you find yourself crying uncontrollably several times a day, then you will need to do much more than eat well. Follow the suggestions in the sidebar on pages 213–215. In addition join a support group, solicit help from family and friends, and if necessary, seek professional help.

Support Groups

"There are many wonderful things about a support group," said Jill, "but the best, I think, is that the people are like family. We've got a common bond, and we can always call one another just to talk. You don't know how many times that telephone call has saved me from screaming or crying. And sometimes it has allowed me to cry, which was okay too."

Like Jill, many caregivers consider their support group as "family." "A place where I can get unconditional love and understanding," "a lifesaver," and "a bright spot in my life" are other comments that describe what support groups mean to their members.

These support groups are formed by family members and other caregivers of people with Alzheimer's who meet for the purpose of offering support and encouragement to each other. They may be run by professionals or experienced caregivers. Many offer information on local resources; some groups share books and other materials with their members. Most of all they are a source of emotional support and friendship. For some caregivers their support-group members are the only "family" they have. They form strong and lasting friendships with other group members, often talking with them on the phone and meeting them away from the group setting.

"Our friends had drifted away one by one," said Larry. "I was alone with Alicia most of the time. When I started going to the support group twice a month, I was amazed at how friendly everyone was. I've made new friends; sometimes a few of us go out for coffee or to a movie after the meeting. Now I have friends I can call and who call me and we understand each other. I don't feel so alone anymore."

Your local Alzheimer's Association office or hospital social worker can give you the location of groups near you.

Family and Friends

Family and friends may feel uneasy around a person who has Alzheimer's, and around you as well.

"Our friends stopped calling," said Natalie. "And I was so tired from taking care of Ron all day that I didn't make the effort to call them. One day I realized I hadn't talked to anyone all week except once to the next-door neighbor. But if I call my friends, maybe they'll feel obligated to come over, and I know Ron makes them feel uncomfortable."

Because family members and friends may not know what to say or may not understand all you're going through, they may stay away. However, that doesn't mean they don't care about you. Often it's up to you to stay in touch. Call your silent family and friends and let them know you need to talk.

"It's good just to have someone to talk to about current events, television shows, books, the weather, anything at all," said Rhonda. "My husband can't communicate anymore. I need to talk to at least one person a day on the phone, or I'll go crazy."

Solicit help from others and accept help from those who offer it. Don't feel guilty about "burdening" them. Let family members and good friends know that you'd appreciate some relief. If there are several willing individuals, set up a schedule.

Tammy solicited the help of her daughter and son-in-law. "I didn't know it, but they were just waiting for me to ask for their help. Now my daughter comes every other Saturday morning and stays until late afternoon. Her husband stays with Sid every Wednesday night while I go to choir practice and then again on Sunday mornings for a few hours. I really look forward to that time to myself."

Psychotherapy and Counseling

Sometimes the pressures of caregiving and the complex emotions involved send people into a depression that a support group cannot alleviate. A psychologist, psychotherapist, or other counselor trained in helping caregivers can assist you in sorting through your feelings and dealing with the anger, pain, and confusion you may feel.

Brenda recalls how she felt before deciding to go to a psychotherapist. "I woke up every morning feeling so hopeless and angry. I knew what I had to look forward to—an hour to get Guy up and dressed, another hour to get him to eat, watching his every move all day and all evening. I spent every day trying not to cry or scream at Guy. Then I woke up one night and began to pray that I would die. That's when I knew I needed help."

You may have the option of either individual or group psychotherapy sessions. Group sessions allow you to work on your feelings under the guidance of a psychotherapist while in the company of people who share your situation. Some caregivers are more comfortable with private sessions.

> ## Take Care of Yourself: A Checklist
>
> • *Eat right:* The combination of stress, fatigue, and poor nutrition is a sure recipe for illness.
>
> • *Plan for routine respite:* Whether it's every six weeks or every six months, plan to get away for at an extended time, at least twenty-four hours. Visit a friend or relative; go to the beach or the mountains.
>
> • *Don't give up all your hobbies and interests:* If you like to sew, do it. If you sing in the choir, make arrangements to go. You may have to give up something or make a compromise, but make sure you keep doing activities that make you feel most fulfilled.
>
> • *Use your imagination to relax:* Practice deep-breathing exercises, yoga, or meditation. These are excellent ways of reducing stress. For twenty minutes a day Edith sits quietly and meditates. She visualizes pleasant scenes from her childhood, her college days, and the early days of her marriage. She allows herself to think only of good times.

- *Do something special for yourself:* A bubble bath, massage, a special dessert, a new shirt.
- *Humor is good medicine; remember to laugh:* "I rent the old *Honeymooners* series on video," said Glenn. "It always makes me laugh." Do whatever tickles your funny bone—listen to tapes of Bob and Ray, watch old episodes of *I Love Lucy*, rent videos of your favorite comedians or movies, read humorous stories or essays, go to a funny movie with a friend and laugh together.
- *Find a social outlet:* Attend a class, join a social or church organization, go to a support group.
- *Do volunteer work:* "When one of the women in the support group told me she does volunteer work twice a week, I thought she was crazy," said Arlene. "Then she told me she helped at the children's clinic because she loves children, and I thought, 'I love animals. Why not volunteer at the animal shelter?' So now I do. I go one morning a week, and it makes me feel so good. I've met some wonderful people and I'm making new friends."
- *Don't isolate yourself:* When you can't get out of the house, use the telephone to keep in touch with relatives and friends. Invite people over—friends, neighbors, relatives, your minister. Write letters. Listen to call-in talk-radio shows.
- *Maintain your personal appearance:* If you look good, you'll feel better.
- *Keep a diary or journal:* Write down how you feel each day. Seeing it in black and white can give you a better perspective.
- *Join a support network:* If you have a computer,

> check to see what on-line support groups are available.
>
> • *Seek spiritual guidance:* Many people find prayer comforting.

Ask your physician, nurse, social worker, or Alzheimer's Association representative for the names of professionals who work with the family members of people with Alzheimer's. Also call your local Area Agencies on Aging for information on support services in your community, and consult the organizations listed in the Resource Guide for additional help.

TWELVE

Resource Guide

The following organizations can be helpful resources for caregivers of people with Alzheimer's:

Alzheimer's Association
919 North Michigan, Suite 1000
Chicago, IL 60611-1676
(800) 272-3900
(312) 335-5776
(312) 335-8882 (TDD)

The Alzheimer's Association is a national voluntary organization that sponsors public-education programs and offers support services to patients and families who are coping with Alzheimer's disease. The organization maintains a twenty-four-hour toll-free hot line and distributes a quarterly newsletter.

Alzheimer's Disease Education & Referral Center (ADEAR)
P.O. Box 8250
Silver Spring, Maryland 20907-8250
(800) 438-4380

This federal organization is a service of the National

Institute on Aging. It provides free brochures, reference materials, and access to a computer database that contains references to recent research and publications on Alzheimer's disease. The center also responds to written and telephone inquiries from health professionals and the public.

American Association of Homes for the Aging
Suite 500
901 East Street, N.W.
Washington, DC 20004-2037
(202) 783-2242

This organization is the national association of not-for-profit organizations dedicated to providing quality housing, health, community, and related services to older people. Free information on long-term care and housing for older people is available to the public (send a self-addressed, stamped envelope).

American Association of Retired Persons (AARP)
601 East Street, N.W.
Washington, DC 20049
(202) 434-AARP

This nonprofit organization sponsors a wide range of educational programs, a computerized bibliographic database, publications, and a mail-order pharmacy.

The American Diabetes Association
1660 Duke Street
Alexandria, VA 22314
(800) 232-3472
(703) 549-1500

This national voluntary health organization supports

diabetes research and education. It offers a toll-free resource number and numerous publications.

American Dietetic Association
Suite 800
216 West Jackson Boulevard
Chicago, IL 60606
(312) 899-0040

The American Dietetic Association is a professional society of dietitians who work in health care settings, schools, day-care centers, business, and industry. Registered dietitians provide nutrition-care services and dietary counseling in health and disease. Many publications are offered, and individuals can call the association to locate a registered dietitian in their community.

American Health Care Association
1201 L Street, N.W.
Washington, D.C. 20005
(202) 842-4444

This professional organization represents the interests of licensed nursing homes and long-term-care facilities to Congress and other groups. Consumers can contact the association for educational materials on long-term care.

American Heart Association
7272 Greenville Avenue
Dallas, TX 75231
(800) 553-6321

This voluntary health organization funds research and sponsors public-education programs to reduce disability and death from cardiovascular diseases and stroke. Free publications are available.

American Occupational Therapy Association
1383 Piccard Drive
P. O. Box 1725
Rockville, MD 20849-1725
(301) 948-9626
(800) 377-8555 (TDD)

This is an organization of professionals who help people with functional problems maintain, increase, or restore their ability to perform daily living skills such as cooking, eating, bathing, dressing, and other activities. Information is available to the public about the role of occupational therapists and local programs.

American Physical Therapy Association
1111 North Fairfax Street
Alexandria, VA 22309
(703) 684-2782

Represents health professionals who help patients recover the greatest possible function following an injury, stroke, or other illness. Physical therapists use exercise, water therapy, and other treatments to strengthen muscles and improve coordination. Individuals can contact the association to learn about qualified physical therapists in their community.

American Psychiatric Association
1400 K Street, N.W.
Washington, DC 2005
(202) 682-6220

A professional society of psychiatrists—medical doctors who specialize in treating people with mental or emotional disorders. Individuals can contact the association to locate a psychiatrist for consultation.

American Psychological Association
750 First Street, N.E.
Washington, DC 20002
(202) 336-5500

A professional society of psychologists—health professionals who counsel people with mental, emotional, or behavioral problems. State chapters help individuals locate a psychologist for consultation and investigate complaints about individual counselors.

American Speech-Language-Hearing Association
10801 Rockville Pike
Rockville, MD 20852
(800) 638-8255

A professional society that distributes a variety of fact sheets on the diagnosis and treatment of speech, language, and hearing disorders. It also has an information helpline that answers questions from the public about communication disorders and offers names of certified audiologists and speech and language pathologists.

Arthritis Foundation
P.O. Box 19000
Atlanta, GA 30326
(800) 283-7800

Nonprofit and voluntary, it offers health education programs and more than one hundred brochures, booklets, videotapes, and other resources for free or minimal cost. Contact your local chapter for a complete listing of materials available or to become a member.

B'nai B'rith International
1640 Rhode Island Avenue, N.W.

Washington, DC 20036
(202) 857-6600

A voluntary service organization that helps people of all faiths. Members of local chapters visit and care for the sick and offer programs to help the poor, older people, and widowed persons.

Catholic Charities USA
Suite 200
1731 King Street
Alexandria, VA 22314
(703) 549-1390

Offers extensive services to older people, including counseling, homemaker services, foster family programs, group homes and institutional care, public-access programs, home health care, health clinics, and emergency assistance and shelter.

Center for the Study of Aging
706 Madison Avenue
Albany, NY 12208-3695
(518) 465-6927

Offers material on aging, health, fitness, and wellness to the public.

Children of Aging Parents (CAPS)
1609 Woodbourne Road
Suite 302-A
Levittown, PA 19057
(215) 945-6900

Provides information and emotional support to caregivers of older persons. It also serves as a national clearinghouse for information on resources and issues dealing with older people. Caregivers nationwide can contact the information and referral service to learn about local resources.

Concerned Relatives of Nursing Home Patients
3130 Mayfield Road
Cleveland Heights, OH 44118
(216) 321-0403

A consumer group that provides information to the public on nursing-home placement and financial assistance. Nursing-home complaints are registered with appropriate regulatory agencies.

Department of Veteran Affairs
Office of Public Affairs
810 Vermont Avenue, N.W.
Washington, DC 20420
(202) 233-5187

Provides benefits to veterans of military service and their dependents. Benefits include educational assistance, home loan programs, and comprehensive dental and medical care in outpatient clinics, medical centers, and nursing homes around the country. Toll-free numbers of VA offices are listed in local telephone directories under "U.S. Government."

Epilepsy Foundation of America (EFA)
4351 Garden City Drive
Landover, MD 20785
(301) 459-3700
(800) 332-1000 (Information/referral only)
(800) 332-4050 (National Epilepsy Library, for professionals)

Offers newsletters, pamphlets, videos, and monographs on epilepsy, as well as the toll-free information hot line.

Foundation for Hospice and Home Care
519 C Street, N.E.
Washington, DC 20002
(202) 547-6586

Promotes hospice and home care, establishes responsible standards of care, and develops programs that ensure the proper preparation of caregivers. Consumer guides, which answer basic questions regarding hospice and home care, are published and distributed free to the public. Individuals can contact the foundation for assistance in locating accredited homemaker-home health services in their area.

Gray Panthers
2025 Pennsylvania Avenue, N.W.
Washington, DC 20006
(202) 466-3132

An advocacy and education group that collects and distributes information about research in the field of aging. An information and referral service offers information to the public about resources for older people.

Health Insurance Association of America
Suite 1200
1025 Connecticut Avenue, N.W.
Washington, DC 20036-3998
(800) 942-4242
(202) 223-7780

Offers information to the public about all aspects of

health and disability insurance. Publications are also available free of charge.

Help for Incontinent People, Inc.
P.O. Box 544
Union, SC 29379
(803) 579-7900
(800) BLADDER (252-3337)

A patient-advocacy group that is a leading source of education, advocacy, and support to the public and to the health profession about the causes, prevention, diagnosis, treatments, and management alternatives for incontinence. A toll-free information service and numerous publications are available.

Legal Services for the Elderly
17th Floor
130 West 42nd Street
New York, NY 10036
(212) 391-0120

An advisory center for lawyers who specialize in the legal problems of older persons also offers a number of publications to the general public.

National Alliance of Senior Citizens
Suite 401
1700 18th Street, N.W.
Washington, DC 20009
(202) 986-0117

A consumer group that provides information to the public about the special needs of older people and about government programs for older Americans.

National Association of Area Agencies on Aging (NAAA)
1112-16th Street, N.W.
Suite 100
Washington, DC 20036
(202) 296-8130

A private nonprofit organization representing the interests of Area Agencies on Aging across the country. Area Agencies on Aging offer such services as transportation, legal aid, nutrition programs, housekeeping, senior-center activities, employment counseling, and information and referral programs.

National Association for Home Care
519 C Street, N.E.
Washington, DC 20002
(202) 547-7424

Distributes information to the public on selecting a home-care agency.

National Citizens' Coalition for Nursing Home Reform
Suite 301
1224 M Street, N.W.
Washington, DC 20005
(202) 393-2018

Sponsors consumer/citizen-action groups around the country that work on behalf of older people and those with disabilities who are institutionalized. Publications are available.

National Council of Senior Citizens
1331 F Street, N.W.
Washington, DC 20004

(202) 347-8800

An advocacy organization of senior activists that works in affiliated local clubs for state and federal legislation to benefit older people and advocate for senior citizens' interests in communities across the United States.

National Council on the Aging, Inc.
409 Third Street, S.W.
Suite 200
Washington, DC 20024
(202) 479-1200

A nonprofit membership organization that provides a national information and consultation service, conducts research, and maintains a comprehensive library of materials on aging.

National Diabetes International Clearinghouse
Box NDIC
9000 Rockville Pike
Rockville, MD 20892
(301) 654-3327

Serves as a centralized resource for information on diabetes and provides consumer and professional publications, a newsletter, and fact sheets.

National Digestive Diseases Information Clearinghouse
Box NDDIC
9000 Rockville Pike
Bethesda, MD 20892
(301) 654-3810

This organization provides information about digestive disease such as diarrhea, heartburn, constipation, and ulcers. Free publications and fact sheets are available.

National Family Caregivers Association
9223 Longbranch Parkway
Silver Spring, MD 20901-3642
(301) 949-3638

A nonprofit membership organization that serves family caregivers and distributes a variety of publications.

National Hospice Organization
Suite 901
1901 North Moore Street
Arlington, VA 22209
(800) 658-8898
(703) 243-5900

This organization provides a referral service and information on hospice services in local areas.

National Institute of Neurologic Disorders and Stroke
Information Office
Building 31, Room 8A06
9000 Rockville Pike
Bethesda, MD 20892
(301) 496-5751

Free publications and information on neurologic diseases, including Alzheimer's and other dementias, are available to the public.

National Institute on Aging Information Center
P.O. Box 8057
Gaithersburg, MD 20898-8057
(800) 222-2225 (Voice)

A federal agency that provides free materials to the public, including fact sheets, pamphlets, and technical reports on Alzheimer's disease, aging research, medical care, nutrition, safety, exercise, and other areas of concern to older adults.

National Kidney and Urologic Diseases Information Clearinghouse
Box NKUDIC
9000 Rockville Pike
Bethesda, MD 20892
(301) 468-8345

Provides information and referrals about products and services related to kidney and urologic diseases.

National Stroke Association
8480 East Orchard Road, Suite 1000
Englewood, CO 80111-5015
1-800-STROKES/(303) 771-1700
Fax: (303) 771-1886

Provides extensive material on stroke prevention, diagnosis, and treatment.

Social Security Administration
Office of Public Inquiries
6401 Security Boulevard
Baltimore, MD 21235
(800) 772-1213
(410) 965-1234

Distributes free publications on benefits and requirements. State Social Security Administration offices are listed in the telephone directory under "Social Security Administration" or "U.S. Government."

United Seniors Health Cooperative
1331 H Street, N.W., #500
Washington, DC 20005-4706
(202) 393-6222

Dedicated to improving the quality and reducing the cost of health and social services for older adults. Members receive counseling on insurance needs, discounts on home-care services and dental care, and referrals to attorneys and mental health providers who specialize in the problems of older people. A variety of publications are also available.

United Way of America
701 North Fairfax Street
Alexandria, VA 22314-2045
(703) 836-7100

An association of local independent agencies in cities and towns across the United States that support social service and public assistance programs, including a variety of community programs for older adults. Local agencies are listed in the telephone directory.

Visiting Nurse Association of America
3801 East Florida Avenue
Suite 206
Denver, CO 80210
(800) 426-2547

Offers information and referrals for home health care services, including physical therapy, occupational therapy, speech therapy, and general nursing. Operates adult-day-care centers, wellness clinics, hospices, and Meals on Wheels programs.

Volunteers of America
3813 North Causeway Boulevard
Metairie, LA 70002
(504) 837-2652

This nonprofit organization offers a variety of social services in communities, including support groups, homemaker assistance, Meals on Wheels, transportation programs, adult day care, group homes for older people, and nursing care.

Glossary

accessibility Refers to the relative ease with which an obstacle (e.g., curb or stair) can be negotiated or a facility or vehicle can be reached or entered by people using crutches, wheelchairs, or who are otherwise restricted in mobility.

adult day care A facility that offers recreational activities and an opportunity for people with Alzheimer's to socialize with other older adults with impairments.

agnosia A perceptual impairment resulting in an inability to recognize familiar objects or associate an object with its use (for example, using a toothbrush to comb one's hair).

Alzheimer's disease A progressive and ultimately fatal neurologic disease that impairs mental function and eventually causes the sufferer to become completely dependent upon caregivers.

atherosclerosis A condition caused by fatty deposits along the inner lining of blood vessels (especially arteries) resulting in narrowing of the vessel and restriction of blood flow.

cardiovascular Refers to heart and blood vessels.

diuretic Type of medication that washes out salt (sodium) from the body and helps to reduce high blood pressure and edema.

durable power of attorney Allows the person with Alzheimer's to select an agent to make all decisions regarding business, property, finances, and so on before he or she is no longer able to make these decisions.

edema Swelling of body parts, due to excessive fluid in the tissue spaces.

foster care A living arrangement that enables some people with Alzheimer's to be cared for in a foster home, where they receive supervision, a room, meals, and transportation to medical facilities.

grab bar A bar, usually metal, solidly fixed to a wall, as in a bathtub, to provide support for people with balance impairments.

health care proxy Allows a person with Alzheimer's to authorize a spouse, adult child, or other adult to make health care decisions for him or her in the event the person becomes mentally incompetent.

hospice A place where individuals who are in the terminal stage of Alzheimer's and have a prognosis of six months or less may live out the remainder of their lives. A hospice offers a caring environment where the person is permitted to die with dignity, and a place where caregivers and their families can receive support and counseling.

hypertension Abnormally high blood pressure; can lead to stroke or heart disease.

incontinence Involuntary discharge of urine or feces.

life-care facility Provides a living situation similar to that of a retirement community; residents receive care for the remainder of their lives, and as their health declines, they are moved to skilled nursing settings within the facility.

living trust Allows people with Alzheimer's to preserve their resources during and after their lifetime. The individual names one or more persons, a bank, or both, as trustee(s).

living will Allows a person with Alzheimer's to clearly state his or her wishes regarding the use of life-sustaining treatment and how health care decisions should be made in the event of mental incapacity.

Medicaid A local health insurance program for people who cannot afford medical and hospital care.

Medicare A federal health insurance program offering hospital and major-medical insurance for disabled people and the elderly.

neurofibrillary tangle An accumulation of abnormal fibers in the nerve cells of the cerebral cortex. Believed to play a role in Alzheimer's disease.

nursing home Also known as a skilled-care facility, this is an alternative living situation for people who need continuous medical and nursing care, including vital-sign monitoring, supervision, administration of medicines, and assistance with daily-living activities.

occupational therapy (OT) Rehabilitation specialty that assists disabled persons to regain or maintain their ability to perform daily activities at home or at work.

physical therapy (PT) Rehabilitation specialty concerned with helping those with impairments from disease, injury, or surgery to restore or maintain functional movement and adapt to permanent disabilities.

plaque A localized abnormal deposit in the brain of a person with Alzheimer's disease.

pressure sore Skin breakdown resulting from prolonged pressure on one spot, usually from sitting or lying in one position too long; also called bedsore or decubitus ulcer.

sliding board A smooth wood or plastic board about two feet long used for transfers of persons unable to stand on at least one lower limb; transfer board.

stroke Sudden loss of function of a part of the brain due to interference in its blood supply.

support group A small group of people who do not have, in this case, Alzheimer's themselves, but who are caregivers or otherwise involved with people with Alzheimer's; its purpose is to provide support and an opportunity for resolving personal concerns, and it is usually coordinated by a counselor or rehabilitation professional.

transfers Movement from one position to another, usually from one seat to another, such as from bed to chair, wheelchair to car, and so on.

Index

Absorbent pads, 83, 86
Accident prevention, 50–51, 70–77
Adaptive devices, 78, 139
Adult day-care centers, 52, 117, 153, 171–174
Aggression, 56–58, 120
Agitation, 26
Agnosia, 124, 134
Alcohol, 60, 61, 118, 120, 146
Allopurinol, 87
Alprazolam, 120
Alternative living arrangements, xviii, 13, 21, 130
  foster care, 174
  hospices, 183
  life-care facilities, 174–175
  nursing homes, 175–181
  state mental hospitals, 181–183

Alzheimer, Alois, 18–19
Alzheimer's Association, 1, 23, 28, 36, 54, 74, 169, 173, 176, 177, 182, 183, 185, 216
Alzheimer's disease
  causes of, 19–21
  communication problems, 31, 33, 40–44
  diagnosis of, 8–9, 21–23
  eating and mealtimes (see Eating; Nutrition)
  exercise (see Exercise)
  financial planning (see Financial planning)
  legal matters (see Legal Matters)
  length of, 9
  living arrangement (see Alternative living arrangements)

Alzheimer's disease *(cont.)*
  medical problems *(see* Medical problems)
  memory loss, xvii, 24, 26, 30–44
  personal hygiene *(see* Personal hygiene)
  personality changes *(see* Mood and behavior problems)
  physical problems *(see* Physical problems)
  prevalence of, xiv
  relationship changes, 10
  social life, 60, 158–161
  symptoms of, 23–24
  treatment, 25–28
Alzheimer's Disease Education and Referral (ADEAR) Center, 19, 216–217
American Association of Homes for the Aging, 217
American Association of Retired Persons (AARP), 217
American Diabetes Association, 128, 217–218
American Dietetic Association, 218
American Health Care Association, 179–180, 218
American Heart Association, 218–219
American Occupational Therapy Association, 218–219
American Physical Therapy Association, 218–219
American Psychiatric Association, 219–220
American Psychological Association, 220
American Speech-Language-Hearing Association, 220
Amitriptyline, 60, 87
Amyloid, 19
Anger, 4, 6, 54, 202, 203–204, 206
Angiotensin converting enzyme (ACE) inhibitors, 127, 128
Antacids, 87
Antianxiety agents, 120
Anticonvulsants, 122
Antidepressants, 51, 60, 118, 119, 133
Anxiety, 4, 26, 46–49, 60, 108
APOE4 (apolopoprotein 4), 20

INDEX

Appetite
 increased, 134
 loss of, 87, 132–134
Arthritis, 77
Arthritis Association, 220–221
Asendin, 119
Atrophy, 156
Attorneys, 17

Bathing, 88–91, 95
Bathroom safety, 74–75, 88
Bedridden, 86, 97, 116, 137
Bedroom safety, 75
Behavior problems (*see* Mood and behavior problems)
Beta-blockers, 127
Biofeedback, 16
Bladder incontinence, 83, 84
Bladder infection, 61, 120
Blood pressure, 12, 108, 109, 127–128, 142, 146
Blood tests, 22
B'nai B'rith International, 221
Body language, 42
Boredom, 50
Bowel incontinence, 83, 85
Brain imaging, 22–23
Brain tumors, 22
Butler, Robert, 38

Caffeine, 49, 118, 148
Calcium channel blockers, 127, 128
Calendars, 35
Calisthenics, 154, 157
Cardene, 128
Cardizem, 128
Car safety, 76
Cataracts, 122
Catholic Charities USA, 221
Center for the Study of Aging, 221
Chewing problems, 109, 136–137
Children, 160–162
Children of Aging Parents (CAPS), 221–222
Chlordiazepoxide, 120
Cholesterol, 144
Cholinergic agonists, 26
Clergymen, 5, 17
Clinging behavior, 58–59
Clinical trials, 27–29, 101, 112
Codeine, 87
Colitis, 133
Combativeness, 10, 24, 31, 54–58, 182
Communication problems, 31, 33, 40–44
Complex carbohydrates, 143
Computerized tomography (CT) scanning, 22–23

Concentration, 59
Concerned Relatives of Nursing Home Patients, 222
Confusion, 10, 24, 26, 34, 46, 60, 129
Conservatorship, 188–189
Constipation, 87–88, 98, 133, 140–143, 152
Consultation appointment, 102
Contact lenses, 124
Contracture, 156
Coordination, loss of, 25, 70, 77–82
Copayment, 195
Coping stage, 5, 7
Counseling, 205, 207, 212–213
Cursing, 55

Daily schedules, 34–35
Dancing, 154, 157
Death, 183
Decision-making abilities, 24
Dehydration, 61, 120, 142
Delusions, 62–63
Denial, 4, 6, 9
Dental care, 16, 98–99, 126
Dentures, 98, 99, 126, 133, 137
Department of Aging, 199

Department of Veteran Affairs, 222
Depression, 4, 6, 12, 22, 26, 31, 59–60, 102, 118, 142, 207
Desipramine, 60
Diabetes, 84, 101, 118, 128, 133, 142, 146
Diagnosis of Alzheimer's disease, 8–9, 21–23
Diarrhea, 140
Dictionary of Medical Specialists, 104
Digestion, 98
Dilantin, 122
Diphenhydramine, 58, 118
Disorientation, 10
Diuretics, 84, 115, 117, 127, 142
Doxepin, 60
Dressing, 55, 91–94
Drooling, 136
Drowsiness, 26
Drug abuse, 61, 120
Drug interactions, 26, 107, 127, 128
Dry mouth, 133
Dry skin, 96
Durable power of attorney, 187, 188

Eating, 25 (*see also* Nutrition)

Eating *(cont.)*
  chewing and swallowing problems, 25, 109, 110, 136–137
  disruptive behavior, 135–136
  inadequate food intake, 132–134
  increased appetite, 134
  successful mealtimes, 138–140
Eating Together Congregate Meals, 198
Edema, 115–116, 117
Elavil, 119
Elimination, 83–86, 90
Embarrassment, 90–91, 203, 208
Emergency assistance, 199
Epilepsy Foundation of America (EFA), 222–223
Estate planning, 192
Exercise, xviii, 60, 87, 108, 117
  in bed, 156–157
  benefits of, 152
  selecting appropriate, 153–155
  tips for regular, 157–158
  wheelchair, 155–156
Eye contact, 43, 56, 139

Falls, 78–79

Familial disease, 20
Family gatherings, 160
Fat, 141, 143–144
Fatigue, 11, 55, 140, 142
Fear, 4, 46, 47, 54
Fecal impaction, 85
Federal Older American Act, 198
Fiber, 87, 109, 141, 143
Fidgeting, 48
Financial planning, xviii, 12, 20–21, 184, 192–200
  calculating cost of care, 193–194
  current financial status, 192–193
  financial assistance, 197–200
  paying for medical care, 194–197
Flash cards, 43
Fluid intake, 83, 85, 87, 141–142
Fluoxetine, 60
Food stamps, 198
Foot care, 97–98
Foster care, 174
Foundation for Hospice and Home Care, 223
Frustration, 6, 31, 55, 202, 203

Genital cleanliness, 90–91

Glasses, 43, 122–124
Grab bars, 74
Grandchildren, 160
Grantors, 189
Gray Panthers, 223
Grieving process, 5–7
Grooming, 94–100
  dental care, 98–99
  foot and nail care, 97–98
  hair, 95
  makeup, 95, 99–100
  shaving, 96
  skin care, 96–97
Guardianship, 188–189
Guilt, 4, 6, 11, 169, 203, 205–206

Hair care, 95
Hallucinations, 26, 61–62, 102, 120
Haloperidol, 58
Headache, 87
Health care proxy, 190
Health Insurance Association of America, 223–224
Health professional team, 14–16
Hearing aids, 43, 125
Hearing problems, 124–126
Heart problems, 20, 60, 118, 133, 143, 146
Heimlich maneuver, 136–137

Helmsley Alzheimer's Alert Program, 53
Help for Incontinent People, Inc., 224
Helplessness, 4, 10
Hoarding and hiding, 64–65
Hobbies, 162–166
Holistic approach, 16
Home-care workers, 90, 169–171
Home-Delivered Meals, 198
Home Energy Assistance program, 199
Hopelessness, 69
Hospices, 183
Hospitalization, 129–130
Humor, 214
Hypertension, 12, 127–128, 142, 146

Ibuprofen, 88, 115
ID bracelet, 53
Identification card, 53
Immune system, 101
Inadequate food intake, 132–134
Incontinence, 25, 26, 83–86, 97
Inderal, 127
Infections, 20, 101
Ingrown nails, 98
Inheritance, 19–20
Injuries, 48, 78–79

INDEX

| 241

Insulin injections, 128
Insurance, 21, 170, 194–197
Internal Revenue Service, 199–200
Irritability, 48

Joint Commission on Accreditation of Hospitals, 179
Judgment, 1, 24
Junk food, 141

Kidney infection, 61, 120
Kitchen safety, 73–74

Language problems, 10
Laxatives, natural, 87
L-deprenyl, 26
Legal matters, xviii, 184–185
　estate planning, 192
　guardianship, 188–189
　health care proxy, 190
　living trust, 189
　living will, 12, 189–190
　power of attorney, 12, 21, 187–188
　"run-ins" with law, 190–191
　wills, 21, 187
Legal Services for the Elderly, 224
Librium, 120
Licensed practical nurses, 15

Life-care facilities, 174–175
Life review, 38
Lifestyle changes, 108–109, 127 (*see also* Exercise; Nutrition)
Life-sustaining measures, 181
Lift transfer, 81, 82
Listlessness, 140, 142
Living arrangements (*see* Alternative living arrangements)
Living trust, 189
Living will, 12, 189–190
Long-term memory, 32, 38

Magnetic resonance imaging (MRI), 23
Magnetic resonance spectroscopy (MRS), 23
Makeup, 95, 99–100
Malnutrition, 140–141
Massage, 96
Masturbation, 67
Meal-preparation tips, 148–149
Meals on Wheels program, 148, 198
Medicaid, 170, 176, 195–196
"Medic Alert" bracelet, 53
Medical history, 21, 22
Medical problems, xvii
　depression, 119–120

Medical problems *(cont.)*
  diabetes, 84, 101, 118, 128
  edema, 115–116
  hearing problems, 124–126
  hospitalization, 129–130
  hypertension, 12, 127–128
  pain, 113–115
  pressure sores, 96–97, 116
  seizures, 121–122
  signs of, 112–113
  sleeplessness, 116–119
  vision problems, 122–124
Medicare, 21, 170, 176, 195
Medications
  knowledge about, 109–110
  organizing, 110–111
  schedule, 12, 13
  side effects of, 26, 60, 107, 111, 114–117, 119–120, 122, 127, 128
Meditation, 16, 26, 60, 108, 213
Memory aids, xvii, 33, 34–35
Memory-enhancement training, 31, 35–36
Memory loss, 24, 26, 30–44
Menu planning, 142–146
Misdirected anger, 204
Mobilization stage, 7

Mood and behavior problems, xvii, 10, 24, 31, 45–68
  anxiety and nervousness, 46–49
  clinging behavior, 58–59
  combativeness, 10, 24, 31, 54–58
  constipation, 87–88
  delusions, 62–63
  depression, 12, 22, 26, 31, 59–60
  hallucinations, 26, 61–62, 102, 120
  hoarding and hiding, 64–65
  medications for, 120
  paranoia, 63–64
  sexuality, 66–68
  wandering and restlessness, 49–54
Music, 49, 56, 59, 85, 115, 118, 139

Nail care, 98
Narcotic analgesics, 114–115
National Alliance of Senior Citizens, 224–225
National Association for Home Care, 225
National Association of Area Agencies on Aging, 225

INDEX

National Citizens' Coalition for Nursing Home Reform, 225–226
National Council of Senior Citizens, 226
National Council on the Aging, Inc., 226
National Diabetes International Clearinghouse, 226
National Digestive Diseases Information Clearinghouse, 227
National Family Caregivers Association, 227
National Hospice Organization, 227
National Institute of Aging, xv
National Institute of Neurologic Disorders and Stroke, 227–228
National Institute on Aging, 228
National Kidney and Urologic Diseases Information Clearinghouse, 228
National Stroke Association, 228
Nervousness, 46–49
Neurofibrillary tangles, 19, 21
Neuroleptics, 77
Neuropsychological tests, 21–22
Nonsteroidal anti-inflammatory drugs (NSAIDs), 115, 133
Nortriptyline, 60
Nurses, 14–15
Nursing homes, 175–181
Nutrition, xvii–xviii, 108
   constipation and, 87
   malnutrition, 140–141
   meal-preparation tips, 148–149
   menu planning, 142–146
   oral hygiene and, 98
   shopping tips, 149–150
   tips for improving, 147–148
Nutritionists, 16

Occupational therapists, 15
Office of Aging, 169, 185
Oral hypoglycemic pills, 128
Organizations, 3, 216–230
Oxazepam, 58

Pacing, 48
Pain, 113–115, 120
Paranoia, 63–64
Parkinson's disease, 77, 84
Partial seizures, 121
Pernicious anemia, 22

Personal hygiene, 12, 13, 25
 bathing, 88–91, 95
 dressing and undressing, 55, 91–94
 grooming (*see* Grooming)
 incontinence, 25, 26, 83–86, 97
 pressure sores, 96–97, 116
Personality changes (*see* Mood and behavior problems)
Pets, 161–162
Pharmacists, 16
 selection of, 107–108
Physical problems, 69 (*see also* Medical problems)
 coordination, loss of, 25, 70, 77–82
 creating safe environment, 70–77
 incontinence, 25, 26, 83–86
 transfers, 81–82
 wheelchairs, 74–76, 79–81
Physical therapists, 15, 106, 169
Physicians, 12, 14
 selection of, 102–106
Physostigmine, 26
Plaques, 19, 21
Pneumonia, 20
Porch and patio safety, 75–76
Positron emission tomography (PET) scanning, 23
Power of attorney, 12, 21, 187–188
Pressure sores, 96–97, 116
Private insurance, 197
Psychiatrists, 16
Psychologists, 16, 106
Psychotherapy, 60, 205, 207, 212–213
Psychotropic drugs, 26

Reaction stage, 6–7
Real estate tax exemption, 199
Reality orientation, 31, 36–38
Recreational activities, 162–166, 171–173
Registered nurses, 15
Relationship changes, 10
Relative responsibility laws, 196
Relaxation exercises, 26
Reminiscence technique, 38–40
Repressed anger, 204
Research studies, 27–29, 101, 121
Resource guide, xviii, 216–230

INDEX

Restlessness, 48, 49–54, 59, 86, 102
Restraints, 129
Retesting, 23
Rocking, 56
Room-by-room safety guide, 73–76

Safety, 70–77, 88
Salt, 145–146
Second opinion, 23
Sectral, 127
Sedatives, 84
Seizures, 121–122
Self-esteem, 36, 38, 92, 94, 100
Senile (neuritic) plaques, 19, 21
Senior Citizen Rent Increase Exemption, 198
Sexuality, 10, 66–68
Shaving, 96
Shock stage, 5–6, 9
Shopping tips, 149–150
Short-term memory, 31–32, 38
Side effects of medications, 26, 60, 107, 111, 114–117, 119–120, 122, 127, 128
Skin care, 96–97
Sleeping pills, 118–119

Sleeplessness, 4, 26, 102, 116–119
Sliding-board transfer, 81
Smoking, 108
Social life, 60, 158–161
Social Security, 198
Social Security Administration, 228–229
Social workers, 5, 15–16, 106, 169
Sodium, 145–146
Spinal fluid, 22
Sporadic, late-onset disease, 20
State mental hospitals, 181–183
Stomach problems, 87, 133
Stress, 19, 23, 28, 209–210, 213
Stroke, 84
Sugar, 141, 142, 144–145
Suicidal thoughts, 59
Supplemental Security Income, 198
Support groups, 3, 5, 70, 207, 210–211
Suspiciousness, 63
Swallowing, 25, 109, 110, 137–138

Tacrine, 26, 111
Tai chi, 16

Taxes, 199–200
Tegretol, 122
Tenormin, 127
Thermometers, 112
Thioridazine, 58
Thyroid problems, 22
Tonic-clonic seizures, 121–122
Tranquilizers, 51, 58, 77, 84
Transfers, 81–82
Trazadone, 118
Tremor, 60
Trusts, 21

Ulcers, 118, 133
Undressing, 91–94
United Seniors Health Cooperative, 229
United Way of America, 229
Urinary incontinence, 83, 84
Urinary tract infections, 84, 118
Urine tests, 22

Velcro closures, 93
Veterans' benefits, 21, 199
Vision problems, 122–124, 133

Visiting Nurse Association of America, 14, 229–230
Visiting-pet program, 162
Visualization, 26, 60, 108, 213
Vitamin B12 deficiency, 22
Volunteers of America, 230

Walking, 153–154
Wandering, 49–54, 152, 190–191
Water
  drinking, 87
  fear of, 54
Wheelchairs, 74–76
  exercises in, 155–156
  ramps for, 80–81
  special features, 79–80
Wills, 21, 187
Withdrawing, 59
Worthlessness, 4

Xanax, 120

Yoga, 16, 26, 60, 213

Marilynn Larkin is an award-winning medical journalist and editor whose articles have appeared in a wide range of national consumer magazines and medical trade publications. She is a contributing editor for **Nutrition Forum**, a former contributing editor for **Health** magazine, and author of three other medical books, including **What You Can Do About Anemia** and **Relief from Chronic Sinusitis** in the Dell Medical Library. Marilynn Larkin lives and works in New York City.